Young People, Physical Activity and the Everyday

Despite society's current preoccupation with interrelated issues such as obesity, increasingly sedentary lifestyles and children's health, there has until now been little published research that directly addresses the place and meaning of physical activity in young people's lives. In this important new collection, leading international scholars address that deficit by exploring the differences in young people's experiences and meanings of physical activity as these are related to their social, cultural and geographical locations, to their abilities and their social and personal biographies.

The book places young people's everyday lives at the centre of the study, arguing that it is this 'everydayness' (school, work, friendships, ethnicity, family routines, interests, finances, location) that is key to shaping the engagement of young people in physical activity. By allowing the voices of young people to be heard through these pages, the book helps the reader to make sense of how young people see physical activity in their lives.

Drawing on a breadth of theoretical frameworks, and challenging the orthodox assumptions that underpin contemporary physical activity policy, interventions and curricula, this book powerfully refutes the argument that young people are 'the problem' and instead demonstrates the complex social constructions of physical activity in the lives of young people. *Young People, Physical Activity and the Everyday* is essential reading for both students and researchers with a particular interest in physical activity, physical education, health, youth work and social policy.

Jan Wright is currently Professorial Research Fellow in the Faculty of Education at the University of Wollongong, Australia.

Doune Macdonald is Professor (Health and Physical Education) and Head of the School of Human Movement Studies at the University of Queensland, Australia.

International Studies in Physical Education and Youth Sport

Series Editor: Richard Bailey

University of Birmingham, UK

Routledge's *International Studies in Physical Education and Youth Sport* series aims to stimulate discussion on the theory and practice of school physical education, youth sport, childhood physical activity and well-being. By drawing on international perspectives, both in terms of the background of the contributors and the selection of the subject matter, the series seeks to make a distinctive contribution to our understanding of issues that continue to attract attention from policy makers, academics and practitioners.

Also available in this series:

Children, Obesity and Exercise
A practical approach to prevention, treatment and management
of childhood and adolescent obesity
Edited by Andrew P. Hills, Neil A. King and Nuala M. Byrne

Disability and Youth Sport
Edited by Hayley Fitzgerald

Rethinking Gender and Youth Sport
Edited by Ian Wellard

Pedagogy and Human Movement
Richard Tinning

Positive Youth Development Through Sport
Edited by Nicholas Holt

Young People's Voices in PE and Youth Sport
Edited by Mary O'Sullivan and Ann Macphail

Physical Literacy
Throughout the lifecourse
Edited by Margaret Whitehead

Muslim Women and Sport
Edited by Tansin Benn, Getrud Pfister and Haifaa Jawad

Physical Education Futures
David Kirk

Young People, Physical Activity and the Everyday

**Edited by
Jan Wright and
Doune Macdonald**

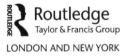

Routledge
Taylor & Francis Group

LONDON AND NEW YORK

First edition published 2010
by Routledge
2 Park Square, Milton Park, Abingdon, Oxon, OX14 4RN

Simultaneously published in the USA and Canada
by Routledge
711 Third Avenue, New York, NY 10017

Routledge is an imprint of the Taylor & Francis Group, an informa business

First issued in paperback 2012

© 2010 selection and editorial material,
Jan Wright and Doune Macdonald; individual chapters, the contributors

Typeset in Times New Roman by Swales & Willis Ltd, Exeter, Devon

British Library Cataloguing in Publication Data
A catalogue record for this book is available from the British Library

Library of Congress Cataloging-in-Publication Data
A catalog record has been requested for this book

ISBN13: 978–0–415–49313–0 (hbk)
ISBN13: 978-0-415-52239-7 (pbk)
ISBN13: 978–0–203–85071–8 (ebk)

Contents

Figures

Contributors

Rebecca Abbott is a Senior Research Fellow in the School of Human Movement Studies at the University of Queensland. Her research focuses on both quantitative and qualitative measurement of children's physical activity and nutrition and its association with health, and she has over 40 peer-reviewed publications and four book chapters in this area.

Matthew Atencio is a postdoctoral research fellow in the Developmental Physical Education Group at the University of Edinburgh. He is interested in researching young people's physical education, health and sport engagements by drawing upon post-structural and post-colonial theories.

Lisette Burrows is an Associate Professor in physical education at the School of Physical Education, University of Otago. Her research is informed by post-structuralist social theory and critical psychology and is focused on the deconstruction of curriculum initiatives, empirical understandings of young people's engagement with physical culture and health and a critical interrogation of developmental discourses in the social construction of formal and informal health and physical education.

Amy S. Ha is Professor and Chair of the Department of Sports Science and Physical Education and the Associate Director of the Center for University and School Partnership at the Chinese University of Hong Kong. Her research interests include critical pedagogy, teacher development and children's physical activity. Over the past years, she had received substantial research grants of Hong Kong and had extensively published her works in both international and regional academic journals.

Kelly Knez holds a research position with the Qatar Orthopaedic and Sports Medicine Hospital, Doha. Her current research is informed by post-structural and post-colonial theory with a particular focus on the intersections between Islam, health, fitness and the body.

Judy Laverty is a senior manager in a government agency responsible for sport, recreation, the arts and social inclusion policy and programmes. She has a background in community development and social policy and recently completed her PhD on meanings of health and well-being amongst young people who have experienced homelessness.

Jessica Lee is a lecturer in physical activity and health at Loughborough University in the School of Sport, Exercise and Health Sciences. Jessica's main research interests lie in the sociocultural understandings of young people's engagements with physical activity and the broader notion of physical culture. She employs a critical sociocultural framework to explore current health and physical activity promotion initiatives and to inform practices that are supportive, equitable and sustainable.

Doune Macdonald is a Professor and Head of the School of Human Movement Studies at the University of Queensland, Australia. Her research interests and work have addressed the challenges of curriculum reform and its impact upon teachers and teaching, and more recently questions of physical activity and young people.

Margaret MacNeill is an Associate Professor at the University of Toronto (Faculty of Physical Education and Health). She is cross-appointed to the Dalla Lana School of Public Health, serves on the Executive Committee for the Collaborative Graduate Program in Women's Health, and is the former Director of the Centre for Research in Women's and Girls' Health and Physical Activity.

Alison Nelson is a doctoral candidate in the School of Human Movement Studies at the University of Queensland. She is also an occupational therapy practice educator and has worked in partnership with an urban Indigenous school for the past 12 years. Alison's research interests are in the area of Indigenous health, and particularly qualitative research exploring perceptions of health and effective health service delivery, areas in which she has published extensively.

Gabrielle O'Flynn is a lecturer in Physical and Health Education in the Faculty of Education at the University of Wollongong. In her research, Gabrielle draws on post-structural theory to critically examine historical and contemporary notions of health and physical activity. Her areas of research include sociological studies of subjectivity in the areas of sport, gender, schooling, physical and health education, and women's health. She has published in journals such as *The British Journal of the Sociology of Education* and *Sport, Education and Society*.

Bonnie Pang is a doctoral candidate in the School of Human Movement Studies at the University of Queensland. She completed her MPhil, which focused on Chinese young people's values in sport, at The Chinese University of Hong Kong. Her current research focuses on the lives of young Chinese immigrants in Brisbane, Australia in relation to their physical activity, health and physical culture.

Geneviève Rail is the Principal of the Simone de Beauvoir Institute, Concordia University, Montreal, Quebec, Canada. She is the Principal Investigator of the Social Sciences and Humanities Research Council of Canada (SSHRC) funded

'*Canadian Youth's Discursive Constructions of Fitness and Health Project*', (Rail, Beausoleil, MacNeill, Burrows and Wright 2003).

Jan Wright is a Professorial Research Fellow in the Faculty of Education at the University of Wollongong. Her research draws on feminist and poststructuralist theory to critically engage issues associated with the relationship between embodiment, culture and health. Her most recent work has focused on social constructions of youth, particularly in the context of public health imperatives and schooling. She is co-editor of *Body Knowledge and Control* (Routledge 2004), *Critical Inquiry and Problem Solving in Physical Education* (Routledge 2004), and *Biopolitics and the 'Obesity Epidemic': Governing Bodies* (Routledge 2009) and co-author with Michael Gard of *The 'Obesity Epidemic': Science, Ideology and Morality* (Routledge 2005).

Acknowledgements

All of the authors in this collection offer their sincere thanks to the many young people who shared their lives and their ideas with us. Thanks also go to their teachers and parents and to the schools who initially provided access to their students.

We also want to express our gratitude to the various funding bodies which supported this research: the Australian Research Council for its six years of funding for the *Life Activity Project*, the Canadian Social Science and Humanities Research Council, Otago University and the Hong Kong Research Council. Special thanks go to Samantha McMahon for her fine eye for detail.

1 Young people, physical activity and the everyday

The *Life Activity Project*

Jan Wright and Doune Macdonald

> I want to achieve a lot with my career and work wise so I know I have to put in the hours but then I feel like I'm missing out on the rest; like the social life, you know, just going for a bike ride, taking the kayak out, motorbike. And when you do think, alright, I've got the time to do it you are just so worn out that you just don't want to do it. It's too much effort. So you just feel tired all the time.
>
> (Karin, Interview *Life Activity Project* 2006)

At first glance, the title of the book is explicit: it looks at young people and the, possibly ordinary, place that physical activity has in their daily lives. However, as this book reveals, for some young people physical activity can bring them regular joy, freedom and sense of accomplishment, while for others, physical activity takes the form of paid work or transport that must be undertaken every day. For yet others, physical activity represents the constant work that must be done on their bodies, in ways that are obligatory and not always pleasurable, to maintain the 'balance' – energy in, energy out – that promises a healthy, slim body. Further, as there are changes in young people's everyday circumstances – a change of school, shifting house, new friends, a part-time job, an injured limb, homework pressures – so too does young people's physical activity participation shift. Curiously, we titled the book before seeing Kenway *et al.*'s (2006: 170) use of the words 'everyday knowledges' which underpin boys' 'reflective self-construction' that is 'situational, temporal and spatial'. We too are interested in young people's reflective self-construction as they take up and resist physical activity each day.

This anthology comprises a set of papers from the researchers involved in the *Life Activity Project* and other projects in New Zealand, Hong Kong, Canada and the United States reflecting its purpose and design. The *Life Activity Project* was motivated in part by the 'moral panic' around young people and the persistent construction of young people, and particularly certain groups of young people, as recalcitrant in their choices around physical activity by dropping out, not being able to 'handle' competition, and becoming sedentary. As researchers working from what might be broadly called a critical sociocultural perspective, we argue that most of the literature on young people and physical activity ignores the complexity and diversity of young people's lives – that is, it fails to take into account how their

choices are made in the context of their personal biographies and the political, economic, cultural and geographical contexts of their everyday lives. The purpose of
the *Life Activity Project* has been to address this gap by documenting the place and
meaning of physical activity in the lives of young people, over time, and across a
wide range of cultural, social and geographical locations.

This chapter will introduce the focus of the book and more specifically outline
the purposes and methodology of the *Life Activity Project*. It also provides an
overview of literature on young people and physical activity from a range of perspectives and, in particular, it will point to the importance of taking account of the
diverse contexts of young people's lives and how their engagement with physical
activity changes over time as their circumstances change. This chapter will conclude with an overview of the book's subsequent sections and chapters to enable the
reader to navigate the book.

The *Life Activity Project*: purpose and methodology

The *Life Activity Project* was originally conceived as a four-year project to investigate the place and meaning of physical activity in the lives of young people from a
range of cultural, social and geographical locations. Further funding from the
Australian Research Council allowed us to extend the project for another three
years and to include groups of young people that we had, in the first four years, been
unable to reach. As a longitudinal study, the *Life Activity Project* makes a third in a
group of Australian studies that have followed cohorts of young people as they
moved through school and beyond. Each of these studies in their different ways
provides insights into the choices, self-perceptions, values and experiences of
young people, as these are influenced by a range of social, cultural and geographic
factors and, as they move through key transitional periods in their lives. Yates and
McLeod's research (The *12 to 18 Project* and the *Transition from School Project*)
has been concerned with how the self-perceptions and social values young people
developed in the contexts of schooling have shaped their aspirations, choices and
experiences in their post-school lives (McLeod and Yates 2006; Yates 1999). In
particular, their work has demonstrated how social class and school contexts, both
within and between schools, are implicated in shaping young people's social values
and expectations in relation to their future career pathways. Coming from a different perspective, Dwyer and Wyn have focused on the fundamental aspects of
change in the relationship between education and employment by following a
cohort of young people through from 1991 to 2004. Through a series of studies,
(*Vocational integration and tertiary education participants of the 1990s* and
*Flexible career patterns: graduate redefinitions of outcomes in the new labour
market*) using surveys and interviews, they investigated the relationship between
young people's expectations and aspirations concerning careers and their actual
career outcomes as they move through school, tertiary study and beyond (Dwyer
and Wyn 2001).

The *Life Activity Project* complements these studies by focusing specifically on
the role of physical activity and related values associated with health as these

contribute to the choices, the self-perceptions and embodiments of young people. Like the aforementioned studies, it followed cohorts of young people as they moved beyond school. The *Life Activity Project* is based on the assumption that longitudinal studies provide essential information about the lives and experiences of a population unavailable from cross-sectional research. It is also based on an assumption that identities and the social and economic circumstances of people's lives are not fixed but neither are lives unaffected by what has come before. It assumes biographies to be produced in relation to changing material and discursive circumstances and that attention to the complex and dynamic nature of lives is necessary to more fully understand how identities are constituted. The chapters in this anthology thus map out young people's changing meanings of health, bodies and physical activity produced in contexts such as schools, families, media, government policy and their changing material circumstances and priorities, such as those associated with geographical location, income, work and relationships.

The research began with a survey of all consenting students (in Australia this meant obtaining parent/guardian consent) in targeted years in eight schools across the three Eastern states of Australia. The schools included: four state-funded high schools, an elite privately funded boys' school and an elite girls' school, a non-elite Catholic high school, and students identified through Queensland's School of Distance Education for remote and isolated children. The survey was adapted from the New South Wales (NSW) Physical Activity Survey (Booth *et al.* 1997) and was designed to provide a demographic snapshot of the schools, the students and their physical activity patterns.

Via the responses to the survey we were able to identify young people from a range of social, cultural and geographical locations for what we called a 'biographical' interview – that is, an interview that took the student through their experiences and engagement with physical activity and physical culture from childhood to the present. The biographical interviews followed a life history approach and asked the young people about their early experiences of physical activity in relation to family, community and school and the influences on their participation and interest in activity. We also asked about their engagement with physical culture more broadly by asking about choices of brand clothing, interest in spectating (live and electronically), in following particular teams and in 2000, their interest and expectations of the Sydney Olympics. On the basis of this interview, we then selected a smaller group of young people who were invited to become participants in a more intensive interview process over the next two years and then with further funding, an additional three years.

The extension of the project in 2004 allowed us to explore young people's meanings of health and physical activity and the shifts in their engagement with physical activity beyond school and in relation to changes in location, income, friendships, family structures and relationships, demands (study, work, church, etc.), and health status. We were able to follow participants through key transitional periods in their schooling, and for some beyond, as these influenced the ways they organized their lives, their relationships, responsibilities and identities around physical activity and leisure. During this period three doctoral students took up specific foci on the intersections of gender and social class (O'Flynn, Chapter 5), gender and geographical location (Lee, Chapter 2) and gender and ethnicity with young Muslim women (Knez, Chapter 8). These students contributed to the data collection across the project but raised specific questions and interviewed and analysed the data of those young people most relevant to their own research. In the second period of the project by involving doctoral students, we were also able to include groups of young people missing from the original research: a cohort of young Indigenous people (Nelson, Chapter 6) and young people who had been homeless (Laverty, Chapter 4).

Data collection

Fifty-four young people (18 primary students, 18 Year 7/8 students and 18 Year 10 students) were chosen across all of the sites to constitute the major cohort group for the *Life Activity Project*. The principal form of data collection was a series of themed interviews with each participant over a two-year period and then follow-up interviews in the ensuing year, with the analysis of initial interviews informing subsequent ones. The first interview revisited the participants' past and present experiences of participation, perceived influences on participation; the second, explored their meanings of health and fitness; and the third, their perceptions of their bodies. For the young women, this usually involved their talking about magazines that they had brought to the interview; for the young men, we developed a series of media photographs of individual and team athletes in various posed and action shots and invited them to talk about these, in relation to their evaluations of the ideal male body. The fourth interview invited participants to use street maps or draw maps to prompt discussions about how they used their local community for leisure and physical activity. These drawings provided rich sets of meanings about important spaces and places in these young people's lives (see Atencio, Chapter 3; Lee and Abbott 2009). Participants were also provided with cameras and asked to take photographs of people and places important to them. This provided a way to explore the place and meaning of physical activity in relation to other aspects of the participants' everyday lives.

In addition to the interviews, the participants were asked to keep ten-day journals, documenting all activities on a daily basis with room for comments (these have provided very interesting insights into the place of school, work, physical activity and other leisure pursuits in the young people's lives). Where possible, the participants were observed engaging in physical activity (within and beyond school) and their feelings about this were discussed in a later interview. The students' physical education and/or class teachers at the project schools were also interviewed about the schools' health and physical education and sport programmes, and related information concerning the practices and values associated with these programmes was gathered.

By the third year of the project (2003) the cohort participants moved into the 'longitudinal' stage of the project; that is, into semi-structured interviews, conducted around the beginning and towards the end of each year. These interviews captured changes in participation patterns, priorities and meanings around physical activity and health and the participants' reflections on what factors relating to schools, communities and families had shaped current behaviours and values. To meet the challenge of following young people beyond school and therefore in many cases out of the family home, the project also explored a range of qualitative methodologies beyond face-to-face interviews such as the use of email, photography, telephone interviews and self-recording on tape in response to a set of questions (already used successfully with students in Jessica Lee's research with rural and isolated young people).

Several other studies drew on the methodology used for the *Life Activity Project*. These included: a study by Lisette Burrows of the meanings of physical activity and health for children in New Zealand (Chapter 12); the meanings of health and fitness for adolescents in a number of Canadian sites conducted by Geneviève Rail and Margaret MacNeill (Chapter 13); and, the place and meaning of physical activity in the lives of young people in Hong Kong, conducted by Amy S. Ha and Bonnie Pang (Chapter 7). Matt Atencio completed his doctoral research by investigating the place and meaning of physical activity in the lives of young people in an inner-city neighbourhood in the United States (Chapters 3 and 11). As is evident from the each of their chapters, these researchers have theorized their data in ways suitable to their context and the questions that motivated their studies.

The analysis of the qualitative data upon which this book draws has taken two main forms: the development of rich contextualized 'stories' for each of the young people in the study; and, a thematic analysis across the data sets using QSR Nvivo. The various researchers have drawn on different social theories depending on their cohort groups, the particular focus of their analysis and their particular chapters. Common across the chapters, and explored in the final chapter of this book, are the researchers' concerns with critical reflection in relation to power and representation in the researcher/researched relationship.

Young people and physical activity: the dominant paradigms

Any database search of young people (or adolescence) and physical activity will produce a flood of articles and reports on young people's physical activity participation: levels of physical activity, motivation to participate, gender and cultural differences in participation and so on (for example, Allen *et al.* 2007; Pate *et al.* 2002). The recent proliferation of these has been largely driven by epidemiological studies of young people's body weight (National Health System 2009; National Preventative Health Taskforce 2009). This research tends to take an instrumental view of 'physical activity', defined as 'any bodily movements performed by skeletal muscles that result in an increase in energy expenditure' (Pink 2008: 2). The range of subcategories falling under this broad definition is outlined below:

> Exercise: Any structured and/or repetitive physical activity performed or practiced where the main intention is to achieve improved physical fitness.
>
> (Pink 2008: 3)

Physical fitness: A set of health (i.e. cardiorespiratory endurance, muscle strength, flexibility) and performance related (i.e. skill, speed, dexterity, mental concentration) attributes that people have in relation to their ability to perform physical activity.

(Pink 2008: 5)

Sport: An activity involving physical exertion, skill and/or eye-hand coordination as the primary focus of the activity, with elements of competition where rules and patterns of behaviour governing the activity exist formally though organizations.

(Pink 2008: 8)

These categories are important because they inform how physical activity can be talked about in research reporting on physical activity, which then informs government policies and interventions. As we demonstrate through our research, it also becomes the way in which young people (and we would argue people more generally) talk about physical activity and attribute value to their own and others' participation. As will become apparent throughout this book, although there is a good deal of slippage in how the young people used these terms, they often narrow how young people talked about physical activity, and contributed to their self-doubt around 'appropriate' physical activity.

Theorizing 'young people'

In the research reported in this collection, we are in part motivated by the need to challenge the deficit model of young people which underpins research on 'declining' rates of participation and consequent increases in the risk to young people's health. Our focus is rather on the young people themselves and how they make sense of physical activity, how it fits into their everyday lives and how and why this might differ for young people from different social, cultural and geographical locations. The *Life Activity Project* is, therefore, informed by an understanding of *youth* as a social process (Wyn and White 1997), that is, one that understands young people's experience to differ historically and for different social and cultural groups. Such a notion of youth also provides a means of conceptualizing transition periods in young people's lives in ways that assume young people's agency and avoid a linear and deterministic approach to development and change. Wyn and White (1997: 77–78) argue that one of the problems with generalizing and universalizing the characteristics of young people is that it serves to 'trivialise and make abstract the lived practices of different categories of youth in ways which distort the social differences and diversity of experience among young people'. They argue for research that will be 'sensitive to the actual lived reality of young people . . . if we are adequately to understand the cultural worlds of the young'. It is this challenge we take up in relation to contemporary young people's experiences of physical activity.

The main alternative thus far to large-scale epidemiological and population studies has been those from sociology of sport and cultural studies, which have investigated young people's engagements with physical culture. These began with research in the 1970s and 1980s in cultural studies departments in the UK that addressed physical activity in the context of particular cultural and subcultural groups. For example, McRobbie's (1984) study of the relationship between dance and fantasy for young women, Brennan's (1993) study of dance and identity and Robbins' (1982) paper on sport and youth culture. More recently and within contemporary understandings of cultural studies, Giardina and Donnelly (2008) have collected a series of papers that critically examine the cultural meanings of sport for young people, in what Denzin's introduction to the book terms 'the historical present'. The 'present' is one characterized by violence, both symbolic and actual violence against children and young people by terrorists, multinationals and agents of the state (including schooling). In their interrogation of 'the articulation of youth sport to culture through a critical cultural studies lens', Denzin (2008: xii) characterizes the authors as engaging in a 'morally centred, politically interventionist project that argues for a politics of truth that answers to enduring issues concerning what is ethical and just'.

In contrast to this mission, our project in this book seems, on the surface, more mundane. Our focus is on individual young people's everyday lives and the place of physical activity in those lives. For some this means engaging in the kinds of youth movement cultures described in the Giardina and Donnelly (2008) collection of papers (for example, Matt Atencio's description of dance, basketball and skateboarding in Chapter 3). For most of the young people in our study, however, physical activity is often an individualized activity and one they fit in around other aspects of their lives. This does not mean that it is not important to their social and cultural identities. It is less likely, however, to take forms that contest or challenge dominant values associated with sport and physical activity. Indeed, one of our questions is to ask why might this be so and what are the implications of this for young people from different social and cultural backgrounds? In this our project is also political. We take as our context the prevailing discourses of health and individual responsibility, and the well-funded campaigns and interventions that disseminate this perspective and act on specific groups of people. We are interested in the kind of citizen subject created by these discourses and how the young people in our study have responded to this (see Chapter 9). We are also interested in challenging a discourse which constantly recites a view of young people as being difficult, deficient and at risk by examining the material conditions of young peoples' lives and their explanations for the place physical activity has in those lives.

From a sociological perspective, a discourse of 'youth at risk' sets up a relationship with young people, which, while it may be well-intentioned, is often adversarial – that is, young people as lacking the capacity to make those decisions that adults believe will make for a better life. At the most extreme, this deficiency is linked to young people's biology, their raging hormones, and most recently the way their brain is wired (Bessant 2008). What such an approach ignores, we would argue, are the complex ways young people negotiate their identities in these particular times. It also ignores how the social and cultural context of the present times impacts on young people's lives and their life chances. For this book, this includes the place and meaning of physical activity in their lives, and the social and cultural contexts which both shape their interest in, but also their opportunities to engage in, physical activity. We argue with McLeod and Yates (2006) and Kenway and her colleagues (Kenway *et al.* 2006) that any investigation of young people's lives must take into account the diversity of their lives and experiences and that this diversity shapes the way they negotiate institutions, relationships and knowledge. We also argue that an analysis of social inequalities is fundamental to an understanding of the 'choices' young people are able to make in their lives. Like the young working-class woman in Walkerdine's (2003) paper, so many of the young people (in the *Life Activity Project*) struggling with making their way, blamed themselves for the 'limited' amount of physical activity in their lives. In this sense they were good moral subjects of a healthism discourse, which lays responsibility with the individual for their health choices and, in the context of our book, their choices around physical activity.

As we demonstrate through our descriptions of young people's everyday lives over time, the choice to be involved in physical activity is rarely one free of constraints; constraints that often flowed from life circumstances that circumscribed their 'choices'. For most of the young people in our study their social, economic and cultural contexts often made it extremely difficult to do the activity they wanted, or believed they needed, to do. As a result, they were left feeling guilty and anxious. It was rare for the young people to interpret their participation in more social terms, far less to attribute their participation choices to structural inequalities.

In making their experiences and their reflections on the place of physical activity in their everyday lives visible through the following chapters, we hope to counter simplistic and universalized deficit versions of young people as making poor choices on the basis of either insufficient knowledge or because of their wanton disregard for the way they are putting themselves 'at risk' of poor future health. The irony is that, for many of the young people, they accept this version of their choices – we hope that by providing another interpretation we may also mitigate some of the guilt and anxiety they feel.

Structure of the book

Cultural geographers, and those in physical activity research drawing on their work, have for sometime pointed to the importance of space as a construct for examining social relations and identities. In Part I of the book, the three chapters in different ways explore the relationships between space, place and individuals' identities/subjectivities. They examine how spaces operate to include and/or exclude the young people in the study and how meanings around health and physical activity are derived from particular uses of urban and rural spaces. In Chapter 2, Jessica Lee, draws on the data from rural young people across the *Life Activity Project* to describe how rural settings, including the institutional setting of the school, shape young people's engagement with and meaning making about physical activity. Matt Atencio, in Chapter 3, uses the data collected for his doctoral study to show how the shared understanding of the hierarchical rankings of basketball courts in parks – in an inner-city neighbourhood, in the United States – served to construct hierarchies of masculinity, which, in turn, worked to exclude those young men (and most young women) who did not measure up. In Chapter 4, Judy Laverty and Jan Wright draw on Life Activity data and data drawn from Laverty's doctoral study to examine how the space of the commercial urban gym influences the way young people in cities organize their lives and manage their identities around health and their bodies.

Part II of the book focuses on the social and cultural locations of young people and how this impacts upon the place and meaning of physical activity. All the chapters in this section drew on the methodology of the *Life Activity Project*, with Chapter 8 a little less so. In Chapter 5, Gabrielle O'Flynn and Jessica Lee use the lens of socio-economic status and its intersection with gender to explore the making of young men and women attending high fee-paying, single-sex, non-government schools in Australia. The lens shifts to Indigenous young people in Chapter 6 led by Alison Nelson with Rebecca Abbott and Doune Macdonald. Nelson *et al.* draw on Critical Race Theory and post-colonialism to decentre 'white ways of knowing' in exploring the intersection of physical activity and sport with the home, family, school and community for urban, Indigenous young Australians.

Chapters 7 and 8 are framed around formal belief systems: Confucianism and Islam. In an increasingly globalized world, it behoves us to better understand how we falsely other and are constructed as Others. Amy S. Ha and Bonnie Pang's research was undertaken with families in Hong Kong in an effort to make explicit the relationships between Confucianism, family practices, and physical activity. In Chapter 8, Kelly Knez shares her participants' stories about being young Islamic women in Australia. The young women talk about their negotiation of physical activity and Islam, the significance of their schools as sites for physical activity and, as with many of the young women across the *Life Activity Project*, the management of their bodies to conform to dominant notions of the ideal.

In Part III the chapters draw on social theory to critically examine the relationship between health, fitness and physical activity. Drawing on data from Life Activity related projects conducted with diverse groups of children and young people, in Australia, New Zealand, Canada and the United States, these chapters each point to the ways moral imperatives associated with health and weight have been taken up or resisted by the participants in talking about their meanings of health. Chapter 9 addresses this issue directly, with Doune Macdonald, Jan Wright and Rebecca Abbott exploring how the imperatives associated with active rational citizenship mesh with young people's ideas and bodily practices in relation to physical activity and health. They conclude by asking whether the very limited resources of contemporary hegemonic health discourses best serve young people in 'knowing' themselves and in becoming (politically) active and informed citizens. In Chapter 10, Jan Wright and Judy Laverty use *Life Activity Project* data (from interviews across the full six-year span of the project) to demonstrate how 'choices' in relation to physical activity change over time and are negotiated in relation to: competing priorities of work and family commitments, as young people move beyond school; and, in relation to their 'physical activity identities', formed in the school years. In Chapter 11, Matt Atencio draws on his interview data, collected in the United States, to examine how young people from different ethnic backgrounds engage with normative ideas about health in both conformist and resistance ways and in so doing construct particular racial and gendered identities. Lisette Burrows' study involved analysing the responses of children from a small, rural town in New Zealand to questions about health in the context of 'childhood obesity' rhetoric. She demonstrates, in Chapter 12, how physical activity was very much part of the children's everyday lives, and how, as 'social actors', they recognized the influence of economic, familial, social and cultural factors on their engagement in physical culture. She argues for more context-specific studies to challenge universalistic (and often deficit) ideas about young people's participation. In Chapter 13, Margaret MacNeill and Geneviève Rail report on data collected from two sites which were part of the larger 'Canadian Youth Constructions of Health and Fitness' Study. They use a post-colonial feminist analysis to explore the ways young people from diverse social and cultural locations make sense of bodily discourses and negotiate practices associated with fitness, nutrition and health.

In our last chapter, Chapter 14, the contributors to the book offer their reflections on methodological issues associated with conducting qualitative research with young people. These include issues of recruiting and maintaining the involvement of the young people, particularly over the longitudinal component of the *Life Activity Project*, and developing respectful relationships which take into account the contexts of young people's lives and cultural sensitivities. The chapter also discusses the dilemmas of (re)presenting the voices and stories of the young people respectfully in research, which for the most part has been informed by a post-structuralist approach that understands stories as fictions associated with particular times and places. In sharing our own stories we attempt to make visible at least some of the 'realities' of doing research with young people, not as confessions, but in the hope that it will be helpful to other researchers working in similar ways with young people.

References

Allen, M., Elliott, M., Morales, L., Diamant, A., Hambarsoomian, K. and Schuster, M. (2007) 'Adolescent participation in preventive health behaviours, physical activity, and nutrition: differences across immigrant generations for Asians and Latinos compared with whites', *American Journal of Public Health*, 97(2): 337–43.

Bessant, J. (2008) 'Hard wired for risk: neurological science, "the adolescent brain" and developmental theory', *Journal of Youth Studies*, 11(3): 346–60.

Booth, M., Macaskill, P., McLellan, L., Phongsavan, P., Okely, T., Patterson, J., Wright, J., Bauman, A. and Baur, L. (1997) *NSW Schools Fitness and Physical Activity Survey, 1997*, Sydney: NSW Department of School Education.

Brennan, D. (1993) 'Adolescent girls and disco dancing', in C. Brackenridge (ed.) *Body Matters: leisure images and lifestyles*, Eastbourne: Leisure Studies Association.

Denzin, N. K. (2008) 'Preface: critical youth studies for the historical present', in M. D. Giardina and M. K. Donnelly (eds) *Youth, Culture and Sport: identity, power and politics*, New York: Routledge.

Dwyer, P. and Wyn, J. (2001) *Youth, Education and Risk: facing the future*, London: Routledge/Falmer.

Giardina, M. D. and Donnelly, M. K. (eds) (2008) *Youth, Culture and Sport: identity, power and politics*, New York: Routledge.

Kenway, J., Kraack, A. and Hickey-Moody, A. (2006) *Masculinity beyond the Metropolis*, New York: Palgrave Macmillan.

Lee, J. and Abbott, R. (2009) 'Physical activity and rural young people's sense of place', *Children's Geographies*, 7(2): 191–208.

McLeod, J. and Yates, L. (2006) *Making Modern Lives: subjectivity, schooling and social change*, Albany, NY: State University of New York Press.

McRobbie, A. (1984) 'Dance and social fantasy', in A. McRobbie and M. Niva (eds) *Gender and Generation*, Basingstoke, UK: Macmillan.

National Health System (2009) *Statistics on Obesity, Physical Activity and Diet: England February 2009*, London: The NHS Information Centre.

National Preventative Health Taskforce (2009) *Australia: the healthiest country by 2020*, Canberra: Commonwealth of Australia.

Pate, R. R., Freedson, P. S., Sallis, J. F., Taylor, W. C., Sirard, J., Trost, S. G. and Dowda, M. (2002) 'Compliance with physical activity guidelines: prevalence in a population, of children and youth', *Ann Epidemiol*, 12(5): 303–8.

Pink, B. (2008) *Defining Sport and Physical Activity: a conceptual model*, Canberra: Australian Bureau of Statistics.

Robbins, D. (1982) 'Sport and youth culture', in J. Hargreaves (ed.) *Sport, Culture and Ideology*, London: Routledge and Kegan Paul.

Walkerdine, V. (2003) 'Reclassifying upward mobility: femininity and the neo-liberal subject', *Gender and Education*, 15(3): 237–48.

Wyn, J. and White, R. (1997) *Rethinking Youth*, Sydney: Allen and Unwin.

Yates, L. (1999) 'Transitions and the Year 7 experience: a report from the 12 to 18 Project', *Australian Journal of Education*, 43(1): 24–41.

Part I

Physical activity and geographical location

2   Focus on the outback

Australian rural young people's diverse experiences of physical activity

Jessica Lee

Introduction and review of literature

Idealized versions of rurality are common throughout the western world. Despite the fact that many people experience rural life differently, the most powerful imaginings of the rural are as a tranquil but hard-working, caring, close-knit community with an open, spacious and safe environment (Valentine 1997). This cultural construction of the countryside, particularly in England, is often termed 'the rural idyll'. More recently, however, it has been acknowledged in academic literature that young people encounter widely disparate experiences and contexts in negotiating rural lives (Panelli 2002). It is therefore important to take account of the 'broader cultural and political processes that shape young people's understandings of rurality and/or their own identit[ies]' (Panelli 2002: 114, note that Panelli originally used the term 'identity'). The purpose of this chapter, then, is to examine, from a sociocultural perspective, the diverse experiences of the Australian rural young people in the *Life Activity Project*, particularly as these relate to their participation in physical activities and their understandings of health and fitness.

Being young in rural Australia

The 'outback' is often described as the 'real' Australia; however, images of rural Australia are contrasting and complicated to say the least. Statistical data depicts rural Australia as having high rates of unemployment, underemployment, poverty and limited economic growth (Bourke and Lockie 2001; Haberkorn *et al.* 2004; Strong *et al.* 1998). For rural young people, research suggests that limited access to good quality health and education services are a particularly important feature of their lives (Quine *et al.*, 2003). From a news media perspective, however, the threat of an 'obesity epidemic' in rural Australia has provided more dramatic headlines. For example, the following headlines appeared after the publication of an article on rural obesity in the *Australian Medical Journal* (Janus *et al.* 2007): 'Rural areas hit hard by obesity' (McLean 2007), 'Obesity "as bad in the bush"' (*ABC News* 2007) and 'Growing concern for fat of the land' (*The Australian* 2007) in the national press. Embedded in the corresponding articles are calls for 'urgent action' by 'increasing physical activity'.

Reporting on the place of physical activity, and particularly sport, in rural Australian communities is also inconsistent. Sport (particularly for men) is often described as the 'social cement' that holds rural communities together (Mugford 2001: 25) and indeed, rural young people have been reported by some sources as just as likely to participate in organized sports as their urban counterparts (e.g. Australian Bureau of Statistics [ABS] 2003). In the past, the popular media has also supported this view claiming on behalf of rural communities, 'We're twice as fit as city kids' (Weston 2004). While studies on physical activity participation of young people in rural Australia are rare, one study suggests that the more geographically remote, the less likely young people were to be physically active (Mummery *et al.* 2000). Conversely, Rossi and Wright (2002) report that parents of isolated rural young people value participation in sports for physical and social development. Internationally, what we 'know' about rural young people's participation in physical activities is also somewhat limited with dated data from the US (e.g. Trost *et al.* 1997) and small qualitative studies from the UK (e.g. Giddings and Yarwood 2005). Due to the lack of organized physical activity options and infrastructure in rural areas (Gard 2001; Mugford 2001; Mummery *et al.* 2000), the school, and in particular Physical Education (PE), has become a space where rural young people can be exposed to, and have the opportunity to participate in physical activities. As such, the approach to PE in rural schools, in particular, can play an important role in shaping young people's engagements with physical activity and physical culture.

The term 'physical culture' has been used in the context of the *Life Activity Project* to signify the ways people speak about their bodies, what they do with their bodies and just as importantly, the silences in their communications; what they do not say or do (Kirk 1999). Associated with this is the identification of those health discourses that shape how people come to understand their bodies. One of the most powerful of these in the contemporary world is a discourse named by Crawford (1980) as 'healthism'. The healthism discourse is the view that health can be achieved 'unproblematically through individual effort and discipline, directed mainly at regulating the size and shape of the body' (Kirk and Colquhoun 1989: 149). The harmful nature of this discourse in school physical education curriculum has been reported, for example in studies which show how young people are uncritically linking body shape to health and fitness (e.g. Burrows *et al.* 2002; Rich *et al.*2004; Wright and Burrows 2004). Reproduction of knowledge and, in particular, the healthism discourse through school PE together with theories of place will be utilized in the following analysis to examine how rural settings (physical and cultural) shape young people's engagements with physical activity and physical culture.

Research method

The 28 young people whose interviews are drawn on for this chapter are those from the *Life Activity Project* (LAP) cohort living in rural locations in two states in Australia: Queensland and Victoria. Participants were recruited from three government schools: Bullion High,[1] in Victoria (15 participants); and, Greenvalley High (eight participants) and Homestead School (five participants), in Queensland. Bullion High is a P-12 school with an approximate enrolment of 300 pupils. The small town of Bullion has a population of around 1,000 and is located 160 kilometres from the state capital. The main industries are dairying, cropping, sheep/wool and beef cattle. Among the cohort of 15 participants (seven male, eight female) some lived in town and others lived on properties. Greenvalley High is a secondary school (approximately 700 students in Years 8–12) in a regional town, in Queensland, located approximately 100 kilometres from the state capital. The town has a population of around 1,000 people, agriculture being the main industry with small farms and acreages. Of the eight participants (five female, three male), some lived in town while others lived on properties up to 30 kilometres from the school.

A further five young people (one female, four male) from Homestead School, a school of distance education, were included in the Queensland cohort. Distance education is a common option in Australia for geographically remote students, where lessons and assessment are conducted via mail, telephone and audiotape with an approved adult (usually the mother) as a home tutor. The five participants lived in four different locations ranging from 250 to 600 kilometres from the capital city. One lived in a small town while the other four lived on more remote properties between 20 and 60 kilometres from the nearest town.

Most interviews were conducted one-on-one and face-to-face either at school or the participant's home; however, participants were offered the choice of convenient venues. Due to the outlying locations of the Homestead School students, some interviews were conducted over the telephone or via audiotape. In addition to participant interviews, three Physical Education teachers from Bullion High and one from Greenvalley High were interviewed on one occasion each. Teachers were asked for their own ideas on health and fitness and about their own school physical education and sports programmes. Participants' parents from all three schools were also interviewed on their own ideas of health and fitness as well as their perceptions of their child's engagements with physical activities.

The findings of this study will be described in two sections exploring the differences and similarities of participants' engagements in physical activities across rural sites/places. The first section is dedicated to exploring the rural young people's participation in physical activities (including sport, recreation, physical labour and Physical Education) and the differences and similarities in these patterns across the different locations. The rural young people's meanings of health and fitness and the role of the healthism discourse in shaping their engagements with physical activities – particularly, within the context of the PE and sport programmes of the respective schools and the views of the PE teachers – is examined in the second section.

Physical activity participation across different rural locations

There are some striking similarities and differences between the Victorian and Queensland rural young people's participation in physical activities. While all of the rural young people talked about participation in recreational physical activities, sports, physical labour and PE, the patterns of engagement between the two states varied. In the case of physical recreation, participation was very similar across the locations. Common examples of activities were walking, jogging and cycling around the property/farm or in the bush, and playing outdoor games or sports with siblings. The following quotes demonstrate how the young people used what was at hand often in very creative ways:

> My golf, I enjoy playing it just down at the paddocks, I think [we have] about 100 acres all up . . . I go for a hit every now and then . . . with my brother, sometimes my dad.
>
> (Henry, Bullion High 2005)

> Well there never used to be grass but we got some rain so it's come up all green so me and [my brother] just used some trees as goals and we play football.
>
> (Jane, Bullion High 2003)

Mouldy: We made a mini golf course.
Int: You and your brothers together?
Mouldy: Yeah . . . we just decided where we were going to put the holes, teed them, then we dug a hole and put a tin in the ground and covered it with some dust so the grass wouldn't grow through it and it's pretty good.

> (Mouldy [male], Homestead School 2002)

> I just do things at home . . . Well, usually if I'm doing anything I go out and talk to my sister who's usually outside on the trampoline. We just start talking and then we go down the road, we go for a walk down the road because there's nothing else to do.
>
> (Jacinta, Greenvalley High 2001)

As evident in these quotes, physical recreation of this type often included family members and was more common amongst the young people in all locations who were more isolated and lived on properties or farms. Interestingly, the rural young people did not describe these physical recreation activities as part of their physical activity but more as part of their general leisure (i.e. they were not mentioned in response to questions about physical activities but in response to others such as 'what else do you do in your spare time?').

In contrast to their participation in physical recreation, participation in sports among the rural young people between the two states was markedly different. The Victorian young people from Bullion High participated in more organized sports than did the Queensland young people from both Greenvalley High and Homestead School. Sports available in the local Greenvalley community were limited to swimming club, golf, touch football tournament and dancing (mostly only catering for primary school girls). A common quote amongst the Greenvalley High participants was that, 'There's nothing to do around here . . . I'd like there to be more things to do' (Jacinta, Greenvalley High 2001).

Sports available in the local towns of the Homestead School participants were similar to (and sometimes more limited than) the ones offered in Greenvalley and due to their mode of schooling they did not have the opportunity to participate in sports teams with the school. They did however participate in some sports:

I'm doing dressage and show jumping and eventing and hacking . . . At the moment I'm working four horses . . . we go to lots of competitions . . . I [also] do highland dancing . . . I do lessons every week and I do an exam or two most years and I go to a few competitions each year.

(Lisa, Homestead School 2002)

The physical activities that I participate in now include club cricket, which I started when I was in Grade 7. My brothers started at the same time . . . It was hard before to do organized sport because we live so far away . . . We don't really go to training because it's an hour away, 52k to go in every Monday night to train.

(Lemming [male], Homestead School 2002)

A larger proportion of Bullion High participants in Victoria, both male and female, were involved in a greater range of sports in comparison to the Greenvalley High and Homestead School participants in Queensland and in sports competition at local, regional and state levels, much of it organized around the school.

We were playing volleyball for our state finals in Melbourne . . . I'm playing cricket with the school and next year I'm doing tennis and dancing.

(Jillian, Bullion High 2003)

Jack: I have arranged to join a [local] athletics club.
Int: How did you get involved in that?
Jack: Well just the school athletics and then we went to [town] for our zones and all won there and just went on from that.

(Jack, Bullion High 2001)

I play netball . . . because they [local league] got an under-15 team up and going, so we play netball and been playing night netball in summer, playing tennis, swimming.

(Janet, Bullion High 2003)

I went along and did some swimming in zone [school rep.] and we've got inter-school netball coming up which is the small schools' cup . . . and we all meet and so we'll play two games of netball and the boys will play footy[2] [Australian Rules]. We've had volleyball already and we've got girls' footy coming up. There'll be soccer towards the end of the year and towards the end of the year there'll also be softball.

(Jeanine, Bullion High 2003)

The range of sports available to the young people from Bullion High, as evidenced in their quotes earlier, is much broader than their peers in Greenvalley through the school or in community clubs, sometimes both. Unlike the Greenvalley participants, the Bullion High young people rarely commented on lack of activities and basketball was the only sport, mentioned by both male and female participants, that was not available in their local area.

What was similar across their participation in both sports and recreational physical activities was the level of family co-participation and support. As mentioned previously, the rural young people commonly participated in physical recreation along with family members. Participants were also involved in sports with their parents and siblings as both co-participants and in other supporting roles, such as transportation.

> I also do horse riding because my dad's an international horse owner. He's been all over the world to design everything. He went to the Olympics to design the courses and everything. My mum was a horse instructor for Greece. She instructed people and helped learn everything for younger kids. The whole family's into horses.
>
> (Henry, Bullion High 2001)

> My dad used to play tennis before he hurt his back and my mum's the president of the tennis club. So she's kind of involved with it . . . and my nan, she plays too. She plays tennis still.
>
> (Janet, Bullion High 2001)

> . . . on Wednesday afternoons if they go to another school because we've got a Tarago [van] kind of thing, we can just about fit the whole [volleyball] team in. So we can take the whole team in one go . . . Transport would be our biggest role, yes.
>
> (Brandon's mother, Greenvalley High 2003)

> I got involved with riding because Mum had horses and she was competing and judging . . . from the start of this year we just dance here at home, in our tiny little lounge room. Mum teaches the dancing . . . six people including me and my sister.
>
> (Lisa, Homestead School 2002)

There was evidence that the strong family influence extended beyond sport into the lives of the rural young people from both states. Due to physical distance and limited structured social opportunities, some of the rural young people spent a lot of time with their families and therefore felt strong family connections. A number of Bullion High young people spoke of following their parents into farming or labour careers, where Greenvalley High and Homestead School participants often saw their parents as inspirational and people whom they admired. '[My role models are] Mum and Dad I guess, just because they work harder than anyone else; that would be the main reason' (Wadiken [male], Homestead School 2003).

Another similarity across the locations was the gendered nature of the participation patterns in sports. The young women who participated in sports remained in *legitimized feminine* activities such as equestrian, tennis, swimming and netball.

Some young women noted the abundance of 'boys'' sports and their lack of access to these: '[the available sports are] based around all boys' stuff . . . they should put more like female sports and stuff' (Sharon, Greenvalley High 1999). Young men in the study also referred to the distinction between *girls'* and *boys'* sports: 'I like playing lots of boys' sports. Some of the girls get annoyed. [Int.: What are boys' sports?] Well like football, cricket, hockey and that' (Mark, Bullion High 2001).

Some flexibility in these gendered norms however, was available for the Bullion High young women, although not without the usual challenges:

> I enjoy football, cricket even though they are boys' games . . . I mean there is nothing wrong with getting the footy and going for a kick.
>
> (Jane, Bullion High 2002)

> Well, I'm sick of every time you go to play football [Australian Rules] it's always the guys who are best. You know, guys do everything but I want to change that so that girls have an equal amount of stuff . . . I've got the back-up [to make up a girls' team] with my dad and my sister . . . some girls think that sport is just for guys. Even though girls play netball and stuff they think there is not a variety of sports to play because guys take over or something. So starting up a football and soccer sort of as a gang or a club sort of thing, it gives the girls time to realize that there's not only netball, [there's] other sports you can do.
>
> (Kim, Bullion High 2003)

It must be noted, however, that these options for the Bullion High young women were generally only available through the school sports programme, which will be discussed further in the following section.

The gender differences observed in the participation in, and perceptions of, physical activity in this study can be placed within a broader gendered social structure. Attribution of responsibility, following traditional gender norms around household chores and childcare, appeared strongly in the interviews both with the rural young people themselves (both male and female) as well as their parents. These trends were consistent across the locations. For example, one Greenvalley High young woman referred to her household chores of 'dishes, washing, mopping, sweeping' as 'woman stuff'. While the young women certainly participated in chores around the farm their input in some areas was restricted, particularly when it came to the more important jobs like driving tractors:

> Well not [my sister], she doesn't drive the tractors . . . only [my brother] and I . . . mainly because I suppose it's sort of rough, it's a boy thing. Like it's not really necessary for her to drive them seeing as [my brother] and I and Dad are all able to.
>
> (Wadiken [male], Greenvalley High 2003)

Int: [looking at photo] Here you are on a tractor and you look like you can drive it, is that true?

Jeanine: Not that one I can't. That's the new tractor, that's my brother's and father's pride and joy, that tractor. It was only bought last year. I haven't been taught to drive that one but I did drive tractors.

Int: So you don't get to drive that one . . .?

Jeanine: That pulls all the big machinery and I'm scared I'd wreck it.

(Jeanine, Bullion High 2003)

For the young women more so than the young men, family responsibilities such as household chores and childcare along with farm chores sometimes restricted their participation in other physical activities. For example, the following were common responses to the question asking what stopped or got in the way of doing physical activity from Bullion High female students: 'My family, I've got a big family and I have to help out a lot' (Jillian, 2003); 'I wanted to go to the football on Friday night but Mum wouldn't let me. I had to stay home and cook Dad's tea' (Sarah, 2002); and '[y]ou can't have too many sports you just don't have time. When we're living on the farm we've got cows to feed, little calves' (Jane, 2001).

In summary, both the Victorian and Queensland cohorts participated in similarly high amounts of recreational physical activities and relied on family support for participation in sports due to distance and travel. However, the Victorian rural young people tended to participate in more sports and have more opportunities to participate than did the Queensland rural young people. Gender differences in participation in sports and physical labour were also noted as similar across both the Queensland and Victorian rural young people. In the next section, the differences and similarities in the rural young people's participation in physical activities (sports and recreation) will be discussed in the context of the PE and sports programmes at their schools.

Physical education and meanings of health and fitness

One of the potential explanations for the differences in participation patterns between the Victorian and Queensland rural young people is the different ways in which they talked about health and fitness. Perhaps the most striking differences in meanings of health and fitness were between the Bullion and Greenvalley High young women. When the young people were asked to define what health and fitness meant to them and why it was important to be healthy and fit (see Chapter 9), the Greenvalley High young women's responses (see following examples) were very strongly embedded in the healthism discourse with frequent reference to the importance of body shape and avoiding 'fatness'.

Sally: Healthy, a lot of exercise, eating good . . .

Int: Why do you think it's important to do more exercise?

Sally: So you don't get fat . . .

Int: Why is it important to be fit?

Sally: So you look good . . . not being big with all these rolls on ya. Just looking slim, looking healthy.

Int:	Is being fit important to you?
Tammy:	No, only image-wise. I don't want to be fat.

Int:	How can you tell if someone is fit?
Sharon:	They just look it, they look really healthy and glowing and muscles, toned.
Int:	Why is it important to be fit?
Sharon:	Because it makes your body look better to be toned.

The Greenvalley High young women tended to see being fit and healthy as related to doing a lot of sport and exercise and the most important outcome of this was to 'look good' or not be 'big/fat'. Interestingly, their concern about body shape and its association with exercise did not translate into high participation rates among the Greenvalley High young women.

The Bullion High young women's views of health and fitness were not totally devoid of talk of body shape; however, they tended to be more interspersed with other meanings such as being healthy to be happy and fit to be better at sports.

Int:	What is the most important part of being healthy for you? What do you get most out of it?
Jeanine:	Always having energy and being happy. There is hardly a day I see myself as not being happy. Like I am always very cheery and my friends always comment on how happy I am. Always ready to run around . . .
Int:	So in terms of fitness what is most important for you about being fit?
Jeanine:	Being able to finish a game of netball successfully . . . not giving up at the start of the last quarter because I am too stuffed. Just being able to play it right through.
Int:	So what is it about healthy food that you are interested in, why are you interested in that?
Jillian:	So if I know what healthy foods to eat I know how to keep fit and so I can keep on playing sports as good as I can.

(Bullion High students 2002)

The meanings of health and fitness for the young men from rural Queensland and Victoria centred mostly around the ability to work and carry out daily tasks and also for sports (see Wright *et al.* 2006). These meanings of health and fitness were played out in their consistent engagements in physical activities including recreation, labour, and sports (see for more detail Lee and Macdonald 2009).

The sources of the young people's knowledge of health and fitness were also an important line of questioning in the *Life Activity Project* in order to understand how dominant discourses, particularly the healthism discourse, were being reproduced. The school, and in particular, Health and PE classes were the most often identified sites of learning for health and fitness knowledge amongst the rural young people in all locations. The school PE and sport programmes and teacher discourses around health and fitness are therefore important sources in helping us to understand the rural young people's understandings of health and fitness and their subsequent participation in physical activities.

Marked differences were noted in the basis of the PE and sports programmes between Greenvalley High and Bullion High. For Greenvalley High the main rationale for the PE programme was health and fitness, for Bullion the emphasis was on social connectedness and personal development. For example, in the following quote the Greenvalley High Health and PE Head of Department (HOD) in describing the focus of the physical fitness stream in the school's PE programme links body shape to fitness in ways that are consistent with the healthism discourse.

> ... fitness does not necessarily mean being a physically fit looking being ... [the PE programme] highlights to them [students] the range of ways you can go about maintaining a reasonable degree of physical fitness so that you're happy with your body and your body shape and size ...
>
> (Greenvalley High, Health and PE HOD 2002)

The way that the Greenvalley High students, particularly the young women, spoke about health and fitness reflected this view of health and fitness. Furthermore, the HOD saw his 'job [as a PE teacher] getting bigger and bigger' as 'obesity is becoming more and more prevalent'. He felt that obesity was a problem at Greenvalley High and that was something of a concern of the school.

Int: Do you feel that with students at your school that there is a problem with obesity?

Teacher: Yes, I think you'd be struggling to find a community that doesn't ... it's still not at an acceptable level. No, obesity even out here, too many kids are overweight, too many kids are I guess not healthy [sic] conscious, which is something we try to change but, as I mentioned earlier, it's a tough job.

> (Greenvalley High, Health and PE HOD 2002)

In contrast to these views, the three PE teachers, including the HOD, from Bullion High who were interviewed, described a focus on in their PE and sports programmes on a socially based curriculum; talk about body shape and obesity were totally absent.

Int: So how important do you think physical activity is in the lives of young people?

Teacher: I think it is very important. As a PE teacher I think it is important and I think it is vital for these kids because sport and physical activity is a real social opportunity in a small town ... the social aspect of sport is an opportunity to learn social skills, all sorts of social skills, just sportsmanship and respect and all those sorts of things.

> (Bullion High, female PE teacher 2005)

Int: When you are constructing a PE lesson with some physical activity in it what becomes a priority for you?

Teacher: Priority would be maximum participation. Getting all the students involved in a lesson and development and learning . . . I try and get kids involved and make it a positive sort of environment for everyone . . .

Int: So what are some of the most important lessons in sport?

Teacher: Just cooperating as a team and doing your best . . . relating to the teachers in a different way [and] with their peers in a different way as well and these are the main lessons I try and encourage. Just participation is important and getting along with everybody.

(Bullion High, male PE HOD 2002)

The differences in approach to PE and sports within the schools can be seen in how the young people themselves from the different schools made sense of health and fitness and engaged with physical activities.

Discussion and conclusion

The findings reported in this chapter have highlighted the diversity of experience among rural young people in Australia. Some experiences in relation to participation in physical activities were similar between the locations, such as a high rate of participation in recreational physical activities particularly for those living on more isolated properties, family involvement and influence, and a gendered notion of what constitutes girls' and boys' activities. However, differences were noted in participation in sports: for example, a larger proportion of the Victorian rural young people, both male and female, participated in a greater range of sports than did the Queensland rural young people. There were also differences in the ways the rural young women talked about health and fitness. The rural young women from Queensland tended to link health and fitness strongly to body shape and appearance, whereas the Victorian young women's meanings of health were more varied and included links to happiness and being fit for sport. These differences in engagements with physical activities and health and fitness discourses may be attributable to differences in PE and sport programme delivery between the schools in the different locations.

Evidence of adherence to gender norms was observed in the current research as the distinction between girls' and boys' sports in both school and club settings was expressed by young people in all locations. This trend is consistent with other research which suggests that the nature of leisure and sports in rural settings tends to follow traditional gender structures (e.g. Dempsey 1992; Henry 1998), such that men's physical activities take precedence over women's and that women can be excluded from participation due to a hegemonic masculine culture. The gendered sport participation patterns are perhaps tied to a more deep seated culture that has been observed in rural Australian communities (see Lee and Macdonald 2009).

The role of family support and co-participation was highlighted in the current findings as important in the rural young people's participation in physical activities, both recreational and organized. Indeed, the importance of the family in the rural context has been identified previously. Sarantakos (1998) claimed that despite the reported challenges faced by rural families, they have been assessed as being as happy as, and functioning as well as, city families. The trends reported in this chapter support the findings of Rossi and Wright (2002) who found that rural and remote families viewed sporting activities as providing social involvement with others.

For rural young people, the school has been identified as an important site for participation in physical activities. This study demonstrated the role of the school context in shaping rural young people's perceptions of health and fitness and participation in physical activities. The dominance of the healthism discourse and its role in the PE curriculum (Azzarito 2007) in shaping young people's perceptions of health and fitness have been previously demonstrated (e.g. Burrows *et al.* 2002; Rich *et al.* 2004; Wright and Burrows 2004). However, the contribution of this chapter is that it demonstrates the differential effect that school PE and sport programmes and indeed perceptions of health and fitness can have on participation in physical activities. Interestingly, the findings reported here are not in the direction that would be anticipated by proponents of an 'obesity epidemic'. Exposure to the healthism discourse and focus on body shape in their school curriculum did not translate into higher participation in physical activities by the Queensland rural young women, although they were indeed well-versed in the discourse. It was the Victorian young people who experienced a more inclusive, socially aware, participation and enjoyment focussed curriculum having more diverse understandings of health and fitness and higher participation in physical activities.

The diversity of experience across the rural locations highlights the importance of place. Australian and international studies tend to concur that rural young people's experiences of place are diverse and strongly influenced by their own interpretations of their social and cultural environments in shaping young people's identities (e.g. Nairn *et al.* 2003; Vanderbeck and Morse Dunkley 2003). A sense of place, including socio-spatial understandings of the intersections of gender and rurality, strong family ties and experiences at school, appears to shape rural young people's perceptions of, and participation in physical activities. It could be argued that the Victorian rural young people's participation in sports was a result of greater access to sporting clubs and local competitions in their own and surrounding towns. Indeed, closure of facilities and lack of interest in local teams was cited by the Queensland rural young people as a barrier to participation. However, the Victorian context may reflect a sociocultural environment valuing participation in sports and leisure activities and thus contributes to the sustainability of such facilities and local competitions. The combination of sociocultural and physical characteristics contributed to a sense of place that was more conducive to participation in physical activities for the Victorian rural young people compared to those from Queensland. These findings highlight the importance of place and importantly that Australian rural young people are a not a homogeneous group, conversely they are exposed to diverse social and cultural circumstances.

This chapter makes several important contributions to the literature on rural young people's understandings of health and fitness and participation in physical activities. First, it highlights the diversity of experience of rural Australian young people and that they should not be considered as a homogeneous group. Second, it describes how rural young people's participation in physical activities is influenced by traditional rural gender roles and the family. Third, it suggests that an inclusive school PE and sport programme focussed on social skills, enjoyment and participation resulted in more diverse understandings of health and fitness and higher participation in physical activities compared to a programme that emphasized body shape and the healthism discourse.

Notes

1 All names of schools, locations and people have been changed to preserve the anonymity of the participants.
2 For the Victorian young people from Bullion High, 'football' or 'footy' refers to Australian Rules football. In Queensland 'footy' can refer to any of three codes, rugby league (most commonly), rugby union or Australian Rules, and so is usually specified. The game of football in the English sense is most commonly referred to as 'soccer'.

References

ABC News (2007) 'Obesity "as bad in the bush"', *ABC News*, 05 August, accessed 15/09/2009, abc.net.au archive.

Australian Bureau of Statistics (2003) *Children's Participation in Cultural and Leisure Activities*, Canberra: Australian Bureau of Statistics.

Azzarito, L. (2007) '"Shape up America!": understanding fatness as a curriculum project', *Journal of the American Association for the Advancement of Curriculum Studies*, 3: 1–23.

Bourke, L. and Lockie, S. (2001) 'Rural Australia: an introduction', in S. Lockie and L. Bourke (eds) *Rurality Bites*, Annandale, NSW: Pluto Press.

Burrows, L., Wright, J. and Jungersen-Smith, J. (2002) '"Measure your belly": New Zealand children's constructions of health and fitness', *Journal of Teaching in Physical Education*, 22(1): 39–48.

Crawford, R. (1980) 'Healthism and the medicalization of everyday life', *International Journal of Health Services*, 10(3): 365–89.

Dempsey, K. (1992) *A Man's Town: inequality between women and men in rural Australia*, New York: Oxford University Press.

Gard, M. (2001) 'Sport, physical education and country towns: diverse enough?', *Education in Rural Australia*, 11(2): 19–26.

Giddings, R. and Yarwood, R. (2005) 'Growing up, going out and growing out of the countryside: childhood experiences in rural England', *Children's Geographies*, 3(1): 101–14.

Haberkorn, G., Kelson, S., Tottenham, R. and Magpantay, C. (2004) *Country Matters: social atlas of rural and regional Australia*, Canberra: Bureau of Rural Sciences.

Henry, J. (1998) 'Bullriding into manhood', in C. Hickey, L. Fitzclarence and R. Matthews (eds) *Where the Boys Are: masculinity, sport and education*, Geelong, Victoria: Deakin Centre for Education and Change.

Janus, E. D., Laatikainen, T., Dunbar, J. A., Kilkkinen, A., Bunker, S. J., Philpot, B., Tideman, P. A., Tirimacco, R. and Heistaro, S. (2007) 'Overweight, obesity and metabolic syndrome in rural southeastern Australia', *The Medical Journal of Australia*, 187(3): 147–52.

Kirk, D. (1999) 'Physical culture, physical education and relational analysis', *Sport, Education and Society*, 4(1): 63–73.

Kirk, D. and Colquhoun, D. (1989) 'Healthism and physical education', *British Journal of Sociology of Education*, 10(4): 417–34.

Lee, J. and Macdonald, D. (2009) 'Rural young people and physical activity: nderstanding participation through social theory', *Sociology of Health and Illness*, 31(3): 360–74.

McLean, T. (2007) 'Rural areas hit hard by obesity', *Herald Sun*, 5 August, accessed 15/09/2007, news.com.au/heraldsun/story/0,21985,22192025-5005961,00.html

Mugford, S. (2001) *The Status of Sport in Rural and Regional Australia: literature, research and policy options*, Canberra: Sport Industry Australia.

Mummery, W. K., Schofield, G. M., Abt, G. and Soper, L. (2000) 'Correlates of adolescent physical activity in regional Australia: results from the Central Queensland adolescent physical activity and nutrition study', paper presented at the AISEP World Sport Science Congress, 2–5 September 2000, Central Queensland University, Rockhampton, Australia.

Nairn, K., Panelli, R. and McCormack, J. (2003) 'Destabalizing dualisms: young people's experiences of rural and urban environments', *Childhood*, 10(1): 9–42.

Panelli, R. (2002). 'Young rural lives: strategies beyond diversity', *Journal of Rural Studies*, 18(2): 113–22.

Quine, S., Bernard, D., Booth, M., Kang, M., Usherwood, T., Alperstein, G. and Bennett, D. (2003) 'Health and access issues among Australian adolescents: a rural–urban comparison', *Rural and Remote Health*, 3 (245), accessed 20/10/2009, http://www.rrh.org.au/publishedarticles/article_print_245.pdf

Rich, E., Holroyd, R. and Evans, J. (2004) '"Hungry to be noticed": young women, anorexia and schooling', in J. Evans, B. Davies and J. Wright (eds) *Body Knowledge and Control: studies in the sociology of physical education and health*, London: Routledge.

Rossi, T. and Wright, J. (2002) 'Children's physical activity, health and physical education in isolated rural contexts: the views of parent educators in Queensland', *Education in Rural Australia*, 12(1): 2–7.

Sarantakos, S. (1998) 'Farm families and city families', in S. Sarantakos (ed.) *Quality of Life in Rural Australia*, Wagga Wagga, New South Wales: Centre for Rural Social Research, Charles Sturt University (pp. 93–103).

Strong, K., Trickett, P., Titulaer, I. and Bhatia, K. (1998) *Health in Rural and Remote Australia*, Canberra: Australian Institute of Health and Welfare.

The Australian (2007) 'Growing concern for fat of the land', 6 August, accessed 15/09/2009, newstext.com.au

Trost, S. G., Pate, R. R., Saunders, R., Ward, D. S., Dowda, M. and Felton, G. (1997) 'A prospective study of the determinants of physical activity in rural fifth-grade children', *Preventive Medicine*, 26(2): 257–63.

Valentine, G. (1997) 'A safe place to grow up? Parenting, perceptions of children's safety and the rural idyll', *Journal of Rural Studies*, 13(2): 137–48.

Vanderbeck, R. M. and Morse Dunkley, C. (2003) 'Young people's narratives of rural–urban difference', *Children's Geographies*, 1(4): 241–59.

Weston, P. (2004) 'We're twice as fit as city kids', *The Sunday Mail*, 18 January, p. 32.

Wright, J. and Burrows, L. (2004) '"Being healthy": the discursive construction of health in New Zealand children's responses to the national education monitoring project', *Discourse: Studies in the Cultural Politics of Education*, 25(2): 211–30.

Wright, J., O'Flynn, G. and Macdonald, D. (2006) 'Being fit and looking healthy: young women's and men's constructions of health and fitness', *Sex Roles*, 54(9–10): 707–16.

3 'I don't wanna die too early'

Young people's use of urban neighbourhood spaces in the United States

Matthew Atencio

Introduction: researching young people's urban neighbourhood spaces

The *Life Activity Project* study in the United States was designed to examine how a group of young people living in a low-income, urban neighbourhood engaged in sport and physical activity. According to Malone (2002: 168) urban neighbourhoods are spaces where the young people who live there gain a 'sense of belonging, place and self-identity through the rituals and "dailyness" of street life'. At the same time, Malone and Hasluck (1998: 26) suggest that young people living in urban neighbourhoods must negotiate 'boundary conflicts' and 'exclusionary practices'. This understanding that urban neighbourhoods contain 'geographies of power' (Malone 2002) which support specific social relations and identities, underpinned my decision to spend three years (2003–6) researching in an adjacent set of urban neighbourhoods located in Mercer City.[1] I had lived near these neighbourhoods prior to the study and I felt that my familiarity with some of the people, sport programmes, streets and parks in this location would provide contacts and information that could help expedite the process of recruiting young people for my study. I eventually moved into the research area and remained there until the end of 2004. During the two years I lived there I was able to observe and interview a group of young people who were engaged in a wide range of physical activities and sports including dance, basketball, soccer, football, running, wrestling, skateboarding and scootering.

I initially attempted to recruit a group of young people from just one neighbourhood. However, it soon became too difficult to find a group of young people who regularly lived within this particular neighbourhood. Many young people in this area lived in several homes (sometimes simultaneously) depending on personal and family situations, financial necessity, and due to sport and physical activity commitments (such as being closer to practice facilities, participating in elite programmes and teams, or training with particular coaches).

The research area that was selected eventually covered four square miles. This area was broad enough to attract a wider number of possible recruits and also incorporated a number of parks, schools and neighbourhoods that were relevant to the young people living in this section of the city. After selecting the research area, I recruited a group of 17 young women and men, aged 13–18, who came from diverse minority-ethnic backgrounds. According to the US Census Bureau (2000), these neighbourhoods have a high population of 'non-Caucasian' residents. They also have a long history of occupation by working class African Americans. High levels of poverty as well as heightened levels of crime and gang activity have impacted these neighbourhoods. For example, between the mid-1980s and early 1990s, they experienced frequent 'gang banging' and high levels of drug dealing and usage. As one writer in a Mercer City newspaper put it:

> In the mid-1980's came King Crack, provider of income, sleek cars, and clothes and an unparalleled high. It was a jobs program for southwest Mercer City the same way it was for South Central Los Angeles and East Oakland. In those days, [two street 'gangs'] set handguns barking against the night.
>
> (*Mercer City News*, 6 September 2000)

Because of the gang scare property prices dropped substantially in the mid-1980s. This changed dramatically in the mid-1990s when the gang problem subsided due to enhanced police efforts, neighbourhood rejuvenation efforts, and increased gentrification of the area. However, there has been a recent resurgence of gang-related shootings and African American and Latino gangs still remain active in the area. Thus, despite recent improvements, life in these neighbourhoods is still challenging.

Young people's sport and physical activity in the Southwest neighbourhoods

The eight young women and nine young men I recruited for the study were aged between 13 and 18 years and came from a range of immigrant and minority-ethnic backgrounds. Three young men were born in Mexico and moved to the United States during primary school. Two young women came from Haiti during middle school and one young woman emigrated from Oromo, a secessionist state within Ethiopia. Eight participants considered themselves to be 'black' or African American. Another young woman described herself as French-Canadian/Hispanic, and two sisters as African American/Cherokee (Native American)/white. Recruitment of these young people occurred in community centres and schools located in the targeted neighbourhoods.

Living in the research area contributed considerably to my knowledge of the young people and their local neighbourhoods. Observations and field notes proved to be very useful means of generating data. Observations involved watching the young people without actively participating in their sport or physical activities. For example, I observed the young people participating in activities such as 'open gym' indoor soccer at Thompson high school, community basketball tournaments in the parks, wrestling clubs, dance recitals, running competitions, skateboarding in the street, and high school football. Notes were taken regarding physical settings, individual and group interactions, specific activities, and young people's behaviour, verbal, and non-verbal communication.

My close proximity to the study participants also provided convenient opportunities to meet with them on a regular basis. Being close to the participants was crucial because it was often difficult to maintain contact because of their various school, work, family, and sport and physical activity commitments. In many instances, their physical activity and sport endeavours were unplanned and I would not know about them until the last minute. For instance, pickup park basketball games could begin at any time during the summer, in numerous locations. Skateboarders might decide on a whim to skate the stairways at the local community college.

Basketball was a very popular and high-profile sport in the study neighbourhoods. There were well-supported basketball camps, open gym programmes, numerous community tournaments, and high school and club teams. Wherever there was an opportunity, young people could often be seen throwing balls up towards portable or makeshift basketball hoops. The larger parks such as Linwood, Willow, Spring and Rafferty were the main spaces where the African American young men in my study played basketball. As I will describe later, the African American young women were rarely able to access these spaces and tended to use local gyms which had organized sessions and adult supervision. Nike refurbished the basketball courts in the neighbourhood parks and these spaces played host to numerous pickup games and community tournaments. Young men, usually white or Hispanic, who rode skateboards and scooters, often used the streets and sidewalks. They also used off-limits spaces such as benches and stair rails found in buildings such as community centres, commercial centres, schools and libraries.

While the young men had access to many of the 'informal' or unsupervised spaces in the neighbourhoods, the young women were more constrained in using these types of spaces due to safety concerns and exclusionary practices enacted by their male peers. Instead the young women used spaces such as gyms and running tracks in situations where coaches or gym supervisors were present. Dancing was also a very popular activity. Many of the Haitian and African American young women talked about dancing in places such as community centres, nightclubs, house parties and even their bedrooms. Thompson high school had several dance studios and offered a dance programme that was nationally recognized; however, many of the African American and Haitian young women felt that this space favoured middle-class, white young women because ballet was a featured activity (see Atencio 2007; Atencio and Wright 2009).

'Social' sport and physical activity spaces

Lefebvre (1991) describes 'spaces' as constitutive of, and constituted by, a nexus of social practices, identities and discourses. Lefebvre proposes that spaces are socially constructed and are contested by those who use them. Furthermore, space, he argues, is both the outcome and the process by which identities, social practices and power relations come to exist. Drawing upon this perspective, van Ingen (2003: 208) suggests that, 'sport landscapes must also be understood as expressions of social relations'. She contends that physical activity and sport spaces support 'multiple relations of domination' structured by 'geographies of gender, sexuality and race' (p. 208).

Following the notion that sport and physical activity spaces are socially constituted and reproductive of hierarchical power relations, I used open-ended interviews and observations to 'map' the young people's engagements with their neighbourhoods. I interviewed the young people in a variety of settings such as a high school office, a pizza shop, the local library and in their homes. Although prepared interview questions were used to guide the interviews, the overall atmosphere was conversational and informal. The majority of interviews took place with individual participants, although some interviews were conducted in pairs and threes when the participants were familiar with each other. Between five and seven interviews per participant took place, and interviews typically lasted between 30 and 60 minutes. The first round of interviews primarily focused on the young people's engagements with health and exercise discourses (see Chapter 10). The second and third rounds of interviews, which inform this chapter, were used to investigate how the young people used their neighbourhood spaces. Later interviews addressed how issues of family, peer groups and popular culture impacted on the young people's sport and physical activity engagements.

During the neighbourhood space interviews, the young people were asked to describe how they moved around and used neighbourhood spaces during a typical week. They were also asked to explain why they used, or did not use, certain spaces, and to describe the people or physical activity programmes that made use of these areas. Photocopies of city maps were used during interviews to help the young people visually reconstruct their various physical activity movements. Visual maps based on templates found on Google Maps and Mapquest were reconstructed to illustrate the young people's physical activity movements during the summer and fall/winter months. Maps were divided according to these two seasons in order to accommodate both school term and summer holiday schedules as well as changes in weather which influenced when outdoor activities and indoor activities were likely to take place. These maps included a range of schools, parks, streets, homes and gyms where the young people engaged in sport and physical activity. I approached the spatial maps as contingently constructed 'texts', which could shed light upon the young people's lives relative to a range of neighbourhood spaces. At the same time, analysing and comparing the individual maps led to a greater understanding of spatial patterns of use that prevailed in particular locations.

The young people's use of neighbourhood spaces

Basketball courts and park spaces

In the Southwest neighbourhoods, Linwood, Spring, Willow and Rafferty parks were known as spaces where pickup basketball could be played. The courts at Rafferty Park were by far the most popular and Spring was sometimes busy; the other parks hosted games on a much more infrequent basis. Rafferty Park's popularity was due, in part, to its recognition as being the most competitive space, hosting 'five on five' pickup games. A local newspaper described Rafferty Park as follows:

> There are plenty of courts in Mercer City for a game of playground basketball, but no blacktop boasts a better caliber of dribble drives, no-look passes and thundering dunks than Rafferty Park . . . Rafferty Park is where those who got game go. If you want to test your skills or just sit back to watch the city's best hoops, this is the place.
>
> (Local newspaper, 21 July 1999)

Fieldnotes indicate that there were three groups of African American young men who played at Rafferty: high school aged players usually affiliated with local high school teams and elite travel teams; 'twenty-somethings' who played at universities and would return on holidays; and older veterans who still lived in the neighbourhoods. In recent years, several players from Rafferty have gone on to play in the National Basketball Association; these players would often return to host charity tournaments or to offer free skills clinics to young people. The five basketball courts at Rafferty would often be filled with players during after-school hours and particularly on Saturday afternoons.

Three African American young men in the study regularly used Rafferty Park: Neal, Jordan and Adam played for the top-ranked Thompson high school team and would come over to Rafferty after school and on the weekends to play. Neal and Adam, in particular, had the capacity to determine access to the park court games and 'shoot arounds', which took place at Rafferty. These two young men were considered by local and even national coaches to be top prospects. By 4:30 p.m. these parks would have 'two courts full' of people playing basketball in 'five on five' games, with large crowds ringing the courts. Because Rafferty Park provided young men such as Neal and Adam with the highest level of competition, it was preferred over other spaces such as Linwood and Spring parks. Jordan, who was a more peripheral member of the high school team and was not as highly regarded as Neal and Adam, had a more difficult time playing games at Rafferty. In all of the parks, including Rafferty, a selection mechanism called 'next' was used to call teams in 'informal' competitive spaces. While pickup games were being played, players who showed up to the court or field called out 'next' to reserve their right to pick teams in the next game. Winners would stay on the court and the new team would be assembled to knock them off the court. Often, there were too many players hanging around the game waiting to be picked, and competition became fierce to get into the games. Those whose abilities were considered inadequate were unlikely to gain 'next' privileges or get picked to play. In these conditions, Jordan mentioned that he could only get 'a game or two' while Adam and Neal said that they could 'run' the games (e.g. remain on the main courts the entire afternoon).

African American young women in the cohort such as Tina and Lorraine had great difficulty accessing the courts at Rafferty when the young men were present (which was often the case). Tina noted that she and her friends were only allowed to shoot around on the side courts that were not being used by the young men: 'we really don't play (games) we just shoot around a lot and work on our shots'. If she was playing a game with other young women, the young men such as Neal and Adam might take the ball and begin taking shots with it. The 'guys' would eventually take over the courts and start playing competitive games. If the young women were initially allowed to play, they would eventually be phased out through 'next' and by practices of intimidation. She later commented that the young women usually ended up watching the young men and then they moved on to a supervised indoor gym to play.

Neal, Adam and Jordan commented that basketball was vital to their everyday survival (e.g. they described it as helping them avoid gang and drug temptations) and to 'making it' out of the neighbourhoods by obtaining university scholarships and even going professional. Finding competitive spaces to 'train' was considered crucial to their basketball development and to gain recognition from local high school and elite travel team coaches. Neal and Adam rarely used spaces such as Linwood, Willow and Spring Park because they thought there was 'no competition' in these spaces; Neal commented that the players in those parks were 'weak'. In comparison, Jordan often used these three parks to play because these spaces hosted less competitive and selective games, and as such, he could 'run' these park court games. After Rafferty, Linwood Park was considered the next best place to play in the Southwest neighbourhoods. Jordan mentioned that this was his neighbourhood park and that his 'boys' would often play there. Local coaches would also go to Linwood to watch and even sometimes play with the high school aged players. Thus, as Jordan noted, it was important to play in the pickup games at Linwood in order to be 'known' as a 'Big Baller'. Linwood had a negative reputation in the Southwest neighbourhoods because fights between gang members would often take place in the park, sometimes on the basketball courts.

The young women in the cohort were particularly wary of playing basketball or doing other physical activity in Linwood. The two Haitian young women, Maureen and Darlene, chose not to go jogging in the park; Maureen commented that there was 'nothing hot' about Linwood and that it was a 'ghetto' and Darlene noted that it was full of 'crackheads' who did nothing but shoot guns and fight all the time.

Spring Park was similarly considered as being a dangerous park for young women and even some of the young men in the cohort. While Jordan would sometimes play basketball games at Spring, this park was mostly avoided by the study participants because it was located on the boundary between two rival gangs. As such, numerous drive-by shootings took place where cars would shoot at suspected gang members 'hanging out' or even playing basketball in the park. The park basketball courts at Spring were covered by a wooden shelter and could appear quite intimidating as it was often dark underneath. Rubee, an East African young woman, said that she did not run in Spring Park because she had heard about the gang shootings which had recently taken place: 'I don't want to be at a park that I'm all by myself, because seven in the morning, you never know who is out there, because a couple be get shot up there'.

Other members of the cohort avoided Spring Park for different reasons. Neal and Adam felt that the competition was 'too weak' and pickup games were too sporadic at Spring. Spring was also considered too far away from where many of the study participants lived; in some instances it was two miles away and many of these young people did not have cars or other means of transport.

Willow Park was similarly linked with gang activity; indeed, one of the local gangs was named after this park. Willow Park hosted infrequent pickup basketball games that were of a low standard, except for Friday nights when local high school players would socialize with friends and play competitive games. Because Willow Park was usually available for basketball, young men such as John would use the courts to play. While the young women in the study tended to avoid Willow because of its dangerous reputation, they did sometimes play games there. However, even in this basketball space, which was relatively peripheral to the local basketball scene, young men such as John would exclude and marginalize the young women. In the following quote, John describes how the young men have 'fun' in Willow Park by playing with the young women and intimidating them by playing 'rough':

Int: What about when the girls play, what is that like?
John: We have fun.
Int: How come?
John: Because they [the 'girls'] would be always talking about don't foul them and [the 'guys'] plays rough with the girls.

(John, interview 2005)

John went on to talk about how the 'guys' would not usually allow the 'girls' to play, since the 'girls' were considered not 'as good as the dudes'.

The exclusion of young women seemed to be standard practice in the parks where basketball took place; 'girls' were considered incapable of handling the physicality of the play. This notion of male 'gatekeepers' who determine access has been noted in other studies of 'open gym' basketball (Wilson *et al.* 2001). In these pickup contexts, young women usually assumed the peripheral role of spectators. The African American young men sustained their dominant positions of power through social practices that devalued the capabilities of and even harmed young women, whom they considered to be physically inferior.

Interviews and observations suggested that the young women predominantly used supervised or organized spaces to conduct their physical activity and sport. Running and playing basketball for the school team or in supervised contexts such as 'all-comers' track meets, in particular, seemed to be safer and more viable contexts for their activities. While the young men seemed to have a wider range of park spaces available to them, young women were mostly constrained from using these public and 'informal' spaces. These findings parallel those of other studies which report women feeling marginalized or at risk in public urban environments, thereby limiting the extent to, and ways in, which they can inhabit these spaces (Domosh and Seager 2001; Watt and Stenson 1998). As a result, many city spaces have been gendered masculine, leading to the continual segregation of city spaces along the lines of 'legitimate' young men and 'illegitimate' young women (Malone 2002). The operation of male power through basketball, coupled with fears of violence and crime, meant that many of the young women in the study became 'illegitimate' users of park spaces.

Street skateboarding spaces

The three Mexican-American young men in the study, Jorge, Elliot and Hector, skateboarded and scootered around much of the research area; riding on streets, curbs, sidewalks, stair rails and benches. Observations and interviews with these young men and others suggested that skateboarding and scootering were growing in popularity in the Southwest neighbourhoods. These activities also seemed to be more socially inclusive activities with different cultural and gender groups represented. A close friend of these young men, who skated with them, was a young white man named Rick, who lived in a different section of the city. Elliot, Jorge and Hector made skate videos which regularly featured young women riding. The young men even noted that a local Brazilian young woman was considered to be the best skateboarder of them all. Skateboarding seemed to be a more social activity compared to basketball and seemed to be an important part of the young men's relationships and friendships with young women. In contrast to other studies (e.g. Atencio *et al.* 2009) the male skateboarders did not exclude female riders by deriding or intimidating them. Unlike pickup park basketball, then, young women were an integral and indeed celebrated part of the street skateboarding culture.

While street skateboarding was a relatively new physical activity in the Southwest neighbourhoods, it was already heavily restricted and given very little community support. Basketball, in both pickup and organized forms, derived considerable support from community groups such as the Salvation Army and the Boys and Girls Club, the local high school, and Nike. In comparison, the young men who participated in skateboarding and scootering had fewer resources and spaces available to them. In her study, Fusco (2007: 53) draws upon Cole's (1996) work to argue that Nike-sponsored facilities are linked with the discourse of white middle-class 'sport, play, health and fitness'. In comparison to sport and fitness, 'street' based activities, such as skateboarding and scooter board riding, seem to be imagined by multinational corporations, communities and schools as less important and even undesirable activities. Although, the very recent sponsorship of urban skate parks by Nike reflects the increasing marketability of this activity, albeit in artificial and controlled urban environments. I argue that the spaces where basketball players played were much more valorized and afforded a much higher cultural status within the neighbourhoods, while skateboarders and scooter riders used marginalized 'street' spaces and were concomitantly positioned quite negatively.

Hector, Elliot and Jorge primarily rode next to a Mexican restaurant; Jorge and Elliot were brothers and worked in this family business. Thus skateboarding and scootering were activities that occurred when they had lunch breaks and when their shift would end. I observed them, along with Hector and Rick, riding in front of the restaurant on makeshift obstacles such as curbs, grates and sidewalks. They made ramps and jumped over hedges located across the street. The young men noted there was a lack of spaces where they could ride in the Southwest neighbourhoods:

Jorge:	... we jump off the curb and ollie over the grate, normally it's like right here [in front of the restaurant] or at Mercer City Community College on the stairs, but we haven't really went to MCCC recently we just kinda skate right there, cos we really got nowhere else to go.
Int:	What do you mean you got nowhere else to go?
Elliot:	If we go over there they might, uh, kick us out and take our boards they're like expensive.

(Jorge and Elliot, interview 2004)

While there were two local skateboard parks approximately five miles away, the young men said they did not use these spaces because they cost money and were often filled with younger kids and their parents. This is very similar to the street skateboarders in Snow's (1999) study who preferred to make their own local and personalized 'spots', from which they gained a sense of belonging. Thus, purpose-built spaces held very little currency, and were 'neither used nor sought after by skateboarders in the same manner as the streets' (p. 22). At the same time, Snow argues that the street skateboarders gained a sense of transgression by using spaces that 'had not been designed to accommodate their needs' (p. 24). As such, street skateboarding has been linked with a form of minority-ethnic masculinity that invokes rebellion, nonconformity and danger (Brayton 2005; Rose and Strike 2004). This desire to take up a subversive masculine identity by using street spaces became even more apparent when Jorge, Elliot and Hector showed me a video tape, in which they had filmed themselves jumping into bushes with their skateboards and scooters and riding in 'off limits' spaces. The young men noted that this behaviour directly mimicked the activities typically found in MTV's *Jackass* series.[2] Arguably, then, these usage patterns in 'off limit' street spaces differentiated Jorge, Elliot and Hector's masculinities from the popular and highly revered basketball players, many of whom considered themselves to be 'role models'. At the same time, street skateboarding gave these Mexican-American young men a sense of belonging in the neighbourhood, as they could use this activity to form supportive relationships with peers from other cultures and genders.

School and free dance spaces

For the young women in the study, dance was a popular and diversified activity. They danced in both institutional settings and 'informal' spaces such as bedrooms, house parties, and nightclubs. Their conversations about dancing provided opportunities to analyse the social practices operating within specific dance spaces. One of the formal and major sites for dance was the dance programme offered at Thompson high school (for more detail, see Atencio and Wright 2009), a public performing and visual arts 'magnet' school. The local students who attended Thompson full-time lived within the school's district boundaries. As such, most of these students were from predominantly African American and lower socio-economic class backgrounds[3] and had no previous formal dance training. During their introductory year, these students were required to take one ballet class for the entire year, supplemented by additional jazz, tap, ballet and African elective classes that each lasted for one semester. In the second year, if the students continued in the dance programme, they took a ballet course that had a small modern dance component for the entire year, and supplemental tap and African class for one semester each.

The full-time, 'local' students who progressed to the third year of the dance programme took tap, ballet and modern. The most advanced and exclusive dance classes were the 'Level Four' classes, which offered ballet, tap and jazz. According to the director, the number of 'local' students diminished as they progressed into the upper-level dance courses. He commented that 'this is where we run into a problem with the dance'. The overwhelming majority of the 'local' students did not make it to the more advanced afternoon classes and the majority of afternoon classes were filled by the more affluent white 'co-op' students who did not attend Thompson full-time. Most of the 'co-op' students came from other Mercer City public high schools and a few of them even came from out of district suburbs and other cities. The primary reason 'co-op' students came to Thompson was because it was renowned for its elite level dance training. In comparison, many of the local young women such as the Haitians, Darlene and Maureen, avoided the programme altogether or quickly dropped out. The emphasis on ballet in the dance spaces was the primary reason for this, as indicated by Darlene in the following quote: 'I never liked ballet anyways, so. Probably why I don't like it now. But . . . hmmm, they tried to have me take and I was like "naww".' Later in the interview Darlene commented that 'I didn't want to do ballet it's too whitey for me. 'Cause I don't like all that music crap: I wanted to take African but I never did.' Other young women also commented that the privileging of ballet in the dance curriculum meant that too much emphasis was placed on maintaining a thin body that resembled white middle-class femininity.

The programme coordinator noted the absence of local young women in the dance programme; indeed, he commented that 5 out of the 60 who started in first year finished the four-year course. I would argue that the local young women were systematically excluded by the structuring of the school dance programme, specifically the mandatory ballet classes in first and second year.

The two young women in the cohort, Sarah and Sasha, who did find value in these dance spaces, even as they were highly critical of the exclusive and segregated nature of these spaces based on race and social class, were from 'mixed white' ethnic backgrounds (French-Canadian/Hispanic and Cherokee (Native American)/African American/white) respectively. Also, these two young women came from more middle-class backgrounds than their more impoverished 'black' peers such as Darlene and Maureen.

Local young women such as Darlene and Maureen often found more value dancing in spaces such as nightclubs, house parties and even in their bedrooms with friends. Indeed, Maureen went to great lengths to describe her love of dancing in a local salsa club. She noted that she would go 'wild' and get 'freaky' in this space and combine elements of hip hop, African and Latin dance styles; she noted that the crowds would wildly cheer on her dancing. The fusional nature of this space contrasted with the more rigid and disciplinary nature of the school dance programme spaces. Even Sasha, one of the young women who came from a more middle-class 'mixed' background and participated extensively in the school dance programme, noted that her involvement in an annual African dance festival was more enjoyable because it was more rhythmic and 'free'. These 'informal' spaces seemed to provide a place where the young women in the study could dance without fear of being excluded, othered and marginalized. At the same time, these spaces catered more directly to their backgrounds in African and hip hop styles of dance and thus provided for more enjoyable and meaningful experiences.

Discussion

In addressing 'social spaces' and gender relations more specifically, Massey (1994) suggests that our understandings of gendered discourses and inequalities can be enhanced by considering the geographic contexts in which they occur. She argues that space shapes gendered social relations. According to Malone (2002), urban neighbourhood spaces create and sustain gendered hierarchies within participants' social worlds. In her interpretation of Sibley's work (1995), Malone defines both 'open' and 'closed' public spaces. Open spaces have weakly defined boundaries, support multiple social and personal values, celebrate difference and diversity, are multicultural, and the policing of boundaries is not necessary in these spaces. Closed spaces have strongly defined boundaries, dominant values are normalized and heavily regulated, difference and diversity are not tolerated, there is a preoccupation with boundary maintenance, high levels of policing exist, and these spaces are typically monocultural.

I argue that closed spaces such as those found in the school dance programme and the park basketball courts privileged particular forms of masculinity and femininity, which served to determine spatial patterns of use. The basketball courts were set up to privilege black masculinity in relation to a 'self-empowerment' discourse. The school dance spaces were defined according to classical ballet; as such, these spaces worked to reproduce notions of white middle-class citizenship as read through young women's bodies and movements. 'Local' young women were largely excluded through these conditions and were heavily disciplined when they did manage to participate in the programme. Arguably, then, these closed spaces were integrally linked with notions of moral citizenship. Following Fusco (2007), I am left concerned about the ways in which public notions of acceptable citizenship came to impact upon the young people's spatial engagements. In her investigation of Nike's PLAY (Place, Activity, Youth) programme, Fusco illustrates how 'constructions of the new public health in the city are highly spatialized and rely on particular kinds of civic (re)imaginings of youth in urban physical activity space(s)' (p. 47). I suggest that the closed spaces of basketball and school dance were discursively constituted according to the desires of community leaders, schools and corporations such as Nike who advance neo-liberal notions of self-empowerment in urban neighbourhoods.

In contrast to these closed spaces, I would argue that the young men who skateboarded and scootered and the young women who danced in non-curricular spaces engaged with open spaces. Spaces such as streets, sidewalks, nightclubs, bedrooms and house parties became sites of agency where power was negotiated, leading to more egalitarian social relations. While closed spaces have largely worked to contain urban young people 'within spaces that are safe, where it is acceptable to "play"' (Willard 1998: 337–38), these young people used improvisational and fusional urban spaces in ways that directly challenge neo-liberal notions of productive and 'good' citizenship that often work to contain and regulate them. Borden (2001), for instance, has suggested that street skateboarding reflects the desire of male skateboarders to use space to define themselves on their own terms, especially in opposition to a more regulated and productive form of adult masculinity.

By highlighting how minority-ethnic young men and women came to use a range of 'closed' and 'open' neighbourhood spaces – often underpinned by notions of neo-liberal citizenship and, at times, resistance to these norms – I argue that urban physical activity and sport cultures are internally diversified. As such, there is not one discrete and identifiable way in which minority-ethnic young men and women come to engage with their physical activity and sport spaces. Within these spaces there exist complex social relations and hierarchies that are constituted and reproduced, leading to a proliferation of social and cultural identities.

Notes

1 The name of the city where the research study occurred has been changed to protect the anonymity of the participants. I have also changed the names of the local high school, neighbourhoods, newspaper authors, city parks and the study participants to keep them anonymous.
2 *Jackass* was shown on MTV from 2000 to 2002, and featured young white men with skateboarding backgrounds performing various crude and dangerous stunts and pranks.
3 The director of the Thompson dance programme says that the racial/ethnic make-up of the morning students is around 90 per cent African American, 5 per cent Hispanic and 5 per cent Caucasian.

References

Atencio, M. (2007) '"Freaky is just how I get down": investigating the fluidity of black feminine subjectivities in dance', *Leisure Studies*, 27(3): 311–27.
Atencio, M. and Wright, J. (2009) '"Ballet it's too whitey": discursive hierarchies of high school dance spaces and the constitution of embodied feminine subjectivities', *Gender and Education*, 21(1): 31–46.
Atencio, M., Beal, B. and Wilson, C. (2009) 'The distinction of risk: urban skateboarding, street habitus, and the construction of hierarchical gender relations', *Qualitative Research in Sport and Exercise*, 1(1): 3–20.
Borden, I. (2001) *Skateboarding, Space, and the City: architecture and the body*, New York: Berg.
Brayton, S. (2005) '"Black-Lash": revisiting the "White Negro" through skateboarding', *Sociology of Sport Journal*, 22(3): 356–72.
Cole, C. L. (1996) 'American Jordan: P.L.A.Y., consensus, and punishment', *Sociology of Sport Journal*, 13(4): 366–97.

Domosh, M. and Seager, J. (2001) *Putting Women in Place: feminist geographers make sense of the world*, New York: Guilford Press.

Fusco, C. (2007) '"Healthification" and the promises of urban space: a textual analysis of place, activity, youth (PLAY-ing) in the city', *International Review for the Sociology of Sport*, 42(1): 43–63.

Lefebvre, H. (1991) *The Production of Space*, Malden, MA: Blackwell.

Malone, K. (2002) 'Street life: youth, culture and competing uses of public space', *Environment and Urbanization*, 14(2): 158–68.

Malone, K. and Hasluck, L. (1998) 'Geographies of exclusion: young people's perceptions and use of public space', *Family Matters: newsletter of the Australian Institute of Family Studies*, 49: 20–26.

Massey, D. (1994) *Space, Place and Gender*, Cambridge: Polity.

Rose, A. and Strike, C. (eds) (2004) *Beautiful Losers: contemporary art and street culture*, New York: Iconoclast and Distributed Art Publishers, Inc.

Sibley, D. (1995) *Geographies of Exclusion*, London: Routledge.

Snow, D. (1999) 'Skateboarders, streets and style', in R. White (ed.) *Australian Youth Culture*, Hobart: Australian Clearinghouse for Youth Studies.

United States Census Bureau (2000) *United States Census 2000*, Washington DC.

van Ingen, C. (2003) 'Geographies of gender, sexuality and race: reframing the focus on space in sport sociology', *International Review for the Sociology of Sport*, 38(2): 201–16.

Watt, P. and Stenson, K. (1998) 'The street: "it's a bit dodgy around there": safety, danger, ethnicity and young people's use of public space', in T. Skelton and G. Valentine (eds) *Cool Places: geographies of youth cultures*, London: Routledge.

Willard, M. (1998) 'Séance, tricknowlogy, skateboarding, and the space of youth', in J. Austin and M. Nevin Willard (eds) *Generations of Youth: youth cultures and history in twentieth-century America*, New York: New York University Press.

Wilson, B., White, P. and Fisher, K. (2001) 'Multiple identities in a marginalized culture: female youth in an "inner-city" recreation/drop-in center', *Journal of Sport and Social Issues*, 25(3): 301–23.

4   Going to the gym

The new urban 'it' space

Judy Laverty and Jan Wright

Introduction

At a time of increasing hype about the health consequences of obesity, it is unsurprising that 'going to the gym' has become increasingly popular amongst most age groups. Tailored children's gyms for 8 to 14 year olds are being established in some western countries as the new antidote for childhood obesity. Such developments illustrate Fusco's (2007: 46) point that urban spaces are increasingly subjected to neo-liberal ideologies of healthism, active living and consumerism and reflect the overlays and interactions between health and space in neo-liberal cities. At the same time Fusco suggests young people's health geographies are missing from current depictions of life in the city, while van Ingen (2003) also draws attention to the need to better 'narrate' notions of identity and the practices that normalize particular health discourses in the physical activity context.

In this chapter we attempt to present such narrations using interviews with young people across three Australian cities. These interviews were collected for the *Life Activity Project* and as part of a small, related study (Laverty 2008) to explore the intersections between young people's negotiation of local geographies and other aspects of their biographies in shaping notions of 'possibility'. In particular, we focus on how young people from a range of backgrounds talked about physical recreation and the meanings they attributed to this as part of their daily lives. Some of the young people in the studies lived in the inner city, while others lived on the urban fringes. Some came from privileged backgrounds and others from families that struggled economically.

Our attention in this chapter is particularly focused on the role played by the commercial gym to understand how young people, in city contexts, organize their lives and manage their identities around health and their bodies. We chose to focus on the 'gym' because it began to feature as the main space for talk about purposive physical activity for most of the young urban dwellers in the *Life Activity Project*. For some it became a space where they could continue to be involved in physical activity when they could no longer make the commitment to organized sport. For others, it was a new venture into physical activity, made possible by changing relationships and life circumstances; and for still others, it was present in their talk as a potential but not yet realized mechanism for taking more control of their health and their bodies. In contrast, for the young mothers in the Laverty (2008) study, managing daily life with children, mostly without family support was challenging enough and the gym was not even on their 'radar'. Data from the *Life Activity Project* demonstrate that while the gym was construed as a convenient solution to busy lives and a flexible space for physical activity and self-improvement, the commercial gym also represented a mechanism for regulation, through the modelling of self-modification practices linked to neo-liberal notions of the young self (Beck and Beck-Gernsheim 2002). We also argue it is a mechanism for both inclusion and exclusion as young people with the capacity to pay accessed the gym and had a chance to realize the preferred, neo-liberal 'gym' body and the 'goods' that are assumed to follow. Others without this economic capacity were excluded from accessing these goods and the physical activity pleasures and sociality that going to the gym can afford.

In this chapter we use notions of 'space' to reflect this interplay between physical activity, the body and notions of self. We draw on van Ingen's (2003) and Fusco's (2007) analyses to discuss space as relational, symbolic and material, and constructed as both the 'medium and outcome of social relations' (van Ingen 2003: 204). As pointed out by Fusco, notions of space are closely aligned to the current discussions of 'place', where power relations play out over spatial dimensions. In using such notions, it is possible to understand how the gym has become a space where health discourses are concurrently represented, imagined, resisted and/or taken up by young people as they construct multiple and fluid identities.

Theorizing physical activity and the role of the gym

Health maintenance, and by association physical activity, is constructed in current policy contexts as a risk management strategy. Lupton (1997) suggests health is being 'repackaged' as a personal responsibility and individual obligation, which includes the management and minimization of risk through self-monitoring, self-regulation and increasingly self-insurance. In a similar way, Fusco's (2007: 44) exploration of Canadian health policy demonstrates how 'individuals in neoliberal societies are increasingly asked to be concerned with their health and wellbeing', and how physical activity and sports landscapes act as sites for regulation and discipline. Fusco's (2007) analysis in particular illustrates how sports spaces and involvements operate to normalize certain behaviours and engender particular ways of being. At the same time within health/sports policy, young people or 'youth' are often represented in contradictory ways. For example, in Australian policy, young people are often positioned as healthy, productive [future] economic citizens involved in the practising of self-regulating health related practice. Alternatively, they are depicted as disordered, problem children, no longer cute and cuddly and in need of significant intervention and modification.

This contrast in how the young neo-liberal self is described and interpreted has a spatial dimension. For example, Fusco (2007: 55) argues young people's use and access to space is framed in current 'discursive imaginations of youth, health and the city' as being about the dangers of uncontrolled youth deviance and the urgent need to save youth from themselves. She points out that such discourses have the potential to not only inscribe and prescribe 'space' in such a way to engage youth as civic participants, but also to construct 'youth as problem'. In this way discussions of youth, health and the city not only articulate how to be a young citizen in the new public health of the city (Fusco 2007), but also who and what constitutes the undesirable, young urban citizen.

The space of the gym

Much has been written in feminist literature of the place of the commercial gym in contributing to stereotypical notions of the female body as slim, toned and youthful (Featherstone 1991). Since that time the gym has become a diversified space: there are now public and private gyms and commercial gyms, women only gyms, gyms in aquatic centres, hotels and shopping centres; gyms which offer a wide range of activities from yoga, to pump, to weights and aerobics. Gyms have become almost synonymous with machines, so you can now have your own 'gym experience' at home, including a tailored mix of machines and programmes. While gyms are still sites for the kind of extreme bodywork described in studies by Monaghan (2001) and others (Klein 1993; Lowe 1998), the responses of the young people in the *Life Activity Project* demonstrate how the meanings of the gym, and the kind of work that happens in gyms is now much more varied, inclusive and linked to healthism discourses. At the same time gyms have become part of the repertoire of possibilities that people are expected to take up in 'becoming healthy'. As the discourses around weight have come to include 'everyone everywhere' (Burrows and Wright 2007), so too the gym (home or otherwise) has become part of the weekly repertoire for those who want to be active, particularly to maintain or gain fitness and 'keep in shape' (which for many is synonymous). What gyms have to offer now exceeds the simple idea of body shaping. 'Going to the gym' is therefore no longer able to be understood as the practice of someone obsessed with their body. It has become more acceptable for all ages, and if you choose your gym or activity, for all body shapes.

Despite the normalizing of the gym as a more everyday, mainstream experience and space, it could be argued that the gym or fitness centre is still about surveillance, measurement and the disciplining of bodies. Markula and Pringle (2006: 83) demonstrate how through 'their space and exercise practices gyms are designed to discipline . . . bodies towards normalcy', towards the ideal male (increased muscularity) or female (thin and toned) body. At the same time, we would argue that fitness is increasingly being constructed as a mainstream moral responsibility, where going to the gym is in itself a demonstration of a desire to be a good citizen, to achieve and practise individual health responsibilities. For example, in relation to the female body, Markula and Pringle (2006: 83) argue that it 'has come to signify a controlled mind and healthy self-confidence'. The opposite then also holds: the body that is not fit, does not demonstrate its health, and is not a normal body. The imperative to work on the body, and in the case of the young people mentioned in this chapter, to work out at the gym, is one that is either taken up or confessed as an absence – as a practice that should be part of a normal life.

Participants profiled in this chapter

Young participants from the *Life Activity Project* who are featured in this analysis came from five different schools in three different parts of Australia. These schools were: Bloomsbury, an elite independent girls school in a major city (see Melinda, Natalie, Faye and Tomiko's interview texts); Sunnydale, a government school on the urban fringes of a large city (see the texts of Chrissie, Angela, Felicia, Felippe and Steve); Malcos, an elite independent school for boys located in a large Australian city (see Aaron's texts); Seachrist College, a non-elite Catholic high school situated in a regional coastal city (see Rachel's texts) and Mondo High, an inner-city co-educational high school (see Maria and Helena's texts). As indicated in a number of other chapters in this book, we use the elite independent schools as markers of social class, while recognizing some of the young people attending these schools and their families were far from affluent (for example, Tomiko and Melinda). Six young people from the schools in the project (Angela, Felippe, Felicia, Melinda, Faye and Tomiko) were from culturally and linguistically diverse communities. Like many other young people, each one was involved in managing close, but sometimes conflictual, family ties at different stages in the interview process.

Two of the three participants in the Laverty (2008) study (Jane and Alison) also feature in this chapter: these were young women with children living on the urban fringes of a major city. The third participant (Arlie) lived in an inner urban area in semi-supported accommodation for people leaving drug rehabilitation. All three of these young people had been homeless in the 18 months prior to the project interviews.

'In your own time' – the gym as flexible space and mechanism for physical activity

As described in Chapter 10, the juggling of work/study commitments with other social activities and family was a theme that continued for all participants during their last years of school and further intensified in the four to five years immediately after school. What was new about this latter time was the lack of the school structure to define and order young people's daily life. Within the less certain post-school context, 'going to the gym' emerged from the *Life Activity Project* interviews as a relevant activity and destination for young people across socio-economic groups (as defined by school type). However, the meanings assigned to going to the gym varied. For example, the young women from Bloomsbury High had access to more extensive physical activity programmes and resources while at school including a school gym, compared to Sunnydale High. Most of these young women positioned the gym as part of a broader continuum of ongoing physical activity that would be part of their life and available to them over time. Some other young people had already started going to the gym when at school, while others such as Angela (Sunnydale High), talked about the gym as providing a more enabling, less marginalizing physical activity experience, *compared* to school. For example, she describes the difference for her between team sports participation at school and the new-found freedoms associated with 'going to the gym' as follows:

> I think the difference is with the past [at school] there were instructions to follow, rules to follow and you had to keep up with other people's pace as a team. So basically I was a bad member of the team because I was letting everyone slow down. With the gym because I'm doing it individually and I'm doing it on my own and it's easier and that's probably why I enjoy it more, because I don't have anyone yelling at me that I am slowing someone down or I'm not doing this right, I'm not doing that right. So I think that's part of the reason I like it more.
>
> (Angela, interview 2005)

In the following quote, Chrissie (Sunnydale) also reflects on the gym as more self-directed and 'fun' compared to school sports:

> There's nothing I don't like about it [the gym], it's heaps of fun and you can do whatever you want and you go at your own pace and you don't have someone leaning over your shoulder asking you how you are or anything and that's good.
>
> (Chrissie, interview 2001)

Like Angela and Chrissie, others in the study talked about the gym as a convenient and flexible form of physical activity, where you could go when you wanted and as often as you wanted. A workout or class at the gym was seen as easier to fit around work/study schedules than organized team sports. In the following texts Steve, a young man who previously attended Sunnydale High, reflects this view:

> I start work at eight o'clock and I finish by four at the latest. I come home get changed, go to the gym, something that I've just picked up. So yeah I've started going to the gym every single day of the week.
>
> So I can go to the gym, jump on the treadmill for a couple of minutes and then go home.
>
> (Steve, interview 2005)

Like almost all the young women interviewed from Bloomsbury, Natalie had a very planned approach to most aspects of her life particularly career and future. She talked about physical activity as critical to her daily life and her notions of self. In the post-school years she had integrated physical activity into her schedule, going to the university gym when studying and mixing this with jogging and playing soccer with a local team. Over the period of interviews her career had progressed and by the last interview (aged 23) she had bought a unit on the southern outskirts of the city with her long-term boyfriend. While Natalie experienced a knee injury and struggled with the realities of her new outer suburban life (commuting, lack of local facilities and absence of street activity at night) she valued her gym membership.

This enabled her to go to gyms in different locations, either close to work or her new home. The gym was a constant in her changed life:

Natalie: I'm going to the gym usually Monday. I do pretty well; I usually go four days a week so I usually go Monday, Tuesday, Wednesday, Thursday after work. So I start work at eight, have a half hour break and finish at four-thirty and then go to the gym for an hour and a half.

Int: Is that here?

Natalie: Yes here. But it is actually really good because it is the same one as in [her new suburb]. So if I don't go after work and I want to go later I can go at [unclear] or if I want to go on Sunday mornings or something, which is good. So start at eight, finish at four-thirty, go to the gym and then go home. I haven't really been doing anything when I get home, you know, just cook dinner, watch TV, that sort of stuff.

(Natalie, interview 2007)

For Melinda, another young woman from Bloomsbury High, the gym provided a more intense physical activity challenge, compared to other options:

I also like the gym because it works more muscles than running does. You know how in running you only work the same muscles all the time or bike riding you work the same muscles. If you go to the gym you can work different muscles and concentrate more on it . . . You have weights and I was trying to work my triceps and I was doing this thing and I wasn't doing it correctly and I had the gym guy fix it up and it hurt like crazy. But at least I'm doing it right, like they've got that method and they've got variety there . . . It's just more of a challenge to me than just running the same path.

(Melinda, interview 2002)

Going to the gym – a normalized site for socializing

While the commercial gym provided convenient, flexible forms of physical activity, some young people in the *Life Activity Project* identified the gym as an important urban space for socializing. 'Gym as social space' was a multiple construction, with young people talking about going to the gym with their friends, current partners or to meet people.

Steve, for example, talked about how the gym had become a central part of his social life:

It [going to the gym] has become a social event as well. You meet lots of people at the gym . . .
. . . physical activity is actually taking a big part of my life now. The gym has become a very social event and I guess that is what keeps me going there as well. We all sit there and while were working out we have this big chat.

(Steve, interview 2005)

And for Aaron, a young man from Queensland (Malcos), going to the gym was synonymous with 'hanging out': 'I like to have a couple of mates over or I go to their place or we head to the gym pretty much. Those are the main places we'll hang out' (Aaron, interview 2006).

For some young people who had been reluctant participants in physical activity at school, the role of friends and particularly the encouragement of partners were important influences. For example, in the following quote, Angela describes how her partner Ahmed was a big influence in her joining the gym:

> Before he [Ahmed] got married he used to go to the gym every second day with his friends. So he just wanted to go back to gym so he was happy to do that. I joined [gym name] and then because Ahmed was doing it so it was good company and so I did it with him . . .
>
> I used to love going to that gym. I mean even if I just spend one and a half hours on it, just going there and coming out I feel really, really good. It's like you feel refreshed, new or something like that, you know what I mean? So yeah I loved going there . . . I think as long as I've got someone there supporting me or pushing me [husband] I am more motivated to do something and I care more . . . So I think other people or friends influence me more.
>
> (Angela, interview 2005)

Unlike most of the other young women interviewed from Bloomsbury, Tomiko had not enjoyed physical activity at school and had spent much more time on her music. However, in 2007 after meeting and moving in with her boyfriend (Josh) she found a new confidence, interest and means of accessing physical activity that she enjoyed. In her last interview when asked about her priorities, she responded:

> Health, physical activity really, yeah those two are at the top of my agenda, which has really changed. Then finances are a bit of a concern because at the moment I just need to get some saving going which I have slacked off a bit and I've kind of decreased my workload to start teaching. So I think I need to build on, preferably teaching but I need to get a bit more money. And yeah, those two. When I say physical activity then it comes hand in hand with Josh so I don't need to put Josh in there I don't think because preferably I would do that with him. So we have a good time when we do something together and it will be that.
>
> (Tomiko, interview 2007)

Family members also played a role in supporting some young people's participation. This included practical support, such as travelling together to the gym, or in terms of exemplifying 'gym going' behaviours. For example, for both Maria (Mondo) and Rachel (Bloomsbury), going to the gym was something they did with their mothers. For Rachel going to the gym was also explicitly explained (with an apologetic laugh) in terms of managing her weight:

Rachel: And some of my friends go.
Int: And that adds more incentive for you.
Rachel: Yeah and my mum goes as well.
Int: Same class or?
Rachel: Yeah, mum does some of the same but she just changed gyms recently.
Int: So is it just to feel better or?
Rachel: Um, I'm very self-conscious about my weight [laughs].

(Rachel, interview 2003)

Constructing notions of self and self-management

Threaded through much of the young people's discussions about going to the gym was the link between their desire to 'feel good about themselves' through managing their weight, building muscle, being fit and capable, and the performance of physical activity. The majority of young women from Bloomsbury, in particular, described how physical activity was an inherent part of their identity, with the gym providing an easily accessible mechanism for practising self-development and body management.

Faye, a young women from Bloomsbury, had described consistently throughout her interviews how important it was to her to do well – academically and in managing her body (see Chapters 9 and 10). The following excerpt, illustrates how, for Faye, her strong work ethic translated into how she felt about her body. The gym provided an individualized mechanism for self-achievement:

> . . . when you usually go and do more physical fitness it's more aimed at a self-goal so in the end what you feel is more self-achievement, in terms of like you've gained more physically, you've actually dragged yourself out to go to the gym to do something by yourself.
>
> It makes you feel better about yourself, and it makes you feel stronger . . .
>
> . . . for example at one point I told you I went to the gym a lot because I think I was feeling a bit restless and I was starting to feel I was getting a bit lazy because I wasn't really doing much like I was sitting around. I think that's when I usually end up not being happy with how I look and I end up thinking that I'm lazy, so that's when I'll go and do something.

(Faye, interview 2002)

Like Faye, Helena, a young women living in Melbourne also talked about the gym as a mechanism for feeling purposeful, productive and looking good:

Int: So what prompted the decision to go to the gym?
Helena: Basically getting in shape for summer and yes just sometimes I have nothing to do after school. I just feel useless so I have to find something to do.

(Helena, interview 2002)

Faye and Helena's descriptions help us to understand how the socially constructed pressure to 'do looks' is internalized and the 'hierarchical valuing of some bodies' (lean, toned and gym styled) over others (larger, less toned and not gym styled) is practised (Frost 2003: 54).

Staying with Faye's account, it is possible to see how over time her notion of self, closely tied to achievement, was strengthened as her career plans firmed up. Faye continued to use physical activity as a way of balancing multiple demands and defining a sense of self-control in her life:

> I think that [physical activity] has always been really important actually, to me sort of, whatever I do. For example with my last job I was working in the city so I joined the gym next door to keep myself busy because I feel that I need to do that every time. I sort of need that balance, otherwise I'm not as happy . . . it just makes me feel better [laughs].
>
> (Faye, interview 2005)

Like Faye, Steve and Melinda talked about physical activity, and in particular the gym, as an 'enabling' mechanism and space, that helped them get 'balance' in their lives.

> My last interview I was managing two of our practices at [city locations] so I was working 140 hour fortnights . . . I was very stressed but it's very much more relaxed now so it's really good and I feel better now by going to the gym and felt that burst of energy . . .
>
> I am really happy that I have made a lot of changes. I would never have gone to the gym or ventured out to find another job but I am really happy that I have.
>
> (Steve, interview 2005)

> In five years time I'll be 23. I'll be finished my degree . . . I'll still be single, not married or anything, because it's too early, work would be very high on my list; very high, because it is sort of like the goal that you've always worked towards . . . Health and stuff I think it's gonna be behind my job, so the job will come first and then maybe going to the gym.
>
> (Melinda, interview 2002)

Faye and to some extent Steve and Melinda's accounts describe the multiple ways that young people integrate and use healthism discourses in their daily lives. Their texts reflect the interaction of neo-liberal notions of individual responsibility, self-management with the enjoyment of physical activity. Their descriptions link body, self and citizenship, and situate and normalize gym life as a core space and activity in their urban lives. The intricacy of these linkages is demonstrated through some young people's descriptions of *not getting to* the gym. Here Melinda and Chrissie describe their sense of disappointment and guilt when not doing (enough) physical activity, emphasizing the strength of 'healthism' as a normalizing discourse:

You can feel it, like you get really flabby after a while . . . you can't do things as quickly and stuff. You feel more tired . . . like I can tell at the moment I'm not doing as much exercise as I should and that's why I feel really mad about it and that's why I want to try going to the gym.

(Melinda, interview 2002)

. . . we used to go to the gym and we used to do the swimming thing but it has completely fallen by the wayside now and I feel so guilty. I think 'ooh I should be doing something'.

(Chrissie, interview 2005)

The gym as an exclusionary mechanism

Within the participant group, access to the gym (that is who could/couldn't go) was in part explained along class lines, with people's participation in the workforce and their capacity to pay being critical influences. While at university and/or in low paid or uncertain employment some young people faced financial pressures. Gym memberships meant the young people often had to make a long-term commitment (e.g. six or twelve months) that was costly. For some getting to the gym was a stop-start activity linked to their changing economic circumstances and work-shifts. Here Angela talks about how access to the gym was closely linked to her job and financial considerations:

Angela: Well before we were members of the gym and then we had to quit because I was [unclear] I quit that job and so there was a financial prob-lem. Then finally now that we have the chance to join in again because we don't have the financial problem, we only have one car between us and I do day shift and he does night shift.

Int: So that is hard to manage that.

Angela: Yes, that's right because he definitely needs the car and the one that I really liked is the one where I started which is in Aqua fitness in Campbelltown and that would be a drive from here.

. . . I know if I join the gym now I would probably just go on Saturdays. So it wouldn't be much point in spending so much money for just that.

(Angela, interview 2005)

The recent trend for local councils to locate gym facilities within multi-purpose aquatic facilities was also highlighted by some young people. For example, the fol-lowing quote is typical of comments from Faye, Melinda and Natalie, who found these facilities to be expensive and less accessible:

I'm in the Sutherland Shire now, I was thinking about joining the Sutherland Aquatic Centre instead of the gym here because you can use the pool as well. But it was about three times as expensive and there [are] not really any other pools. There is one at Caringbah but that is a lot further to go and yeah, there is nothing around near me, there [are] no swimming pools. They do have a fairly new basketball stadium across the road from me but it is mostly kid's sports. . . . I don't know, sometimes it just gets too expensive.

(Natalie, interview 2007)

For some young people living in urban areas 'going to the gym' was talked about as something they would like to do, and which would be a 'good thing' to be able to do, but which they presently could not include in their lives. Here Felippe (Sunnydale), a young man from the outer suburbs of Sydney describes how he wanted to go the gym and had a possible pathway for doing this, but not the commitment at the time:

Probably [I'd rate my health] like a two out of ten; it is not where I want to be like that is another thing I feel like Uni is tying me down because I want to go to the gym or something to do some sort of fitness because one of my work-mates before he goes to work he goes to the gym and then he can have a shower at the office and I was thinking that it's a really good idea just to keep healthy. And I could probably go with him because he just goes to the gym in the city and then he goes to work.

(Felippe, interview 2005)

In later interviews Felippe had more time for physical activity after leaving university. He talked about working out, at home, with his older brother, to increase his weight and build muscle.

Felicia, however, a young woman also from Sunnydale who by the end of the interview period was a young mother with four children, described going to the gym as something she wanted and planned to do in the future. Arguably this was for all kinds of reasons including (but not only) to get back into shape:

Oh yes I plan to do a lot of exercise after the baby is born . . . and book myself in the gym, monthly or three monthly and I can go any day, any time as many times as I want during the day. And right across from the gym is the local swimming pool.

(Felicia, interview 2003)

Later interviews indicate that Felicia never made it to the gym; looking after a home, a baby/children and a partner who worked very long hours were higher priorities.

While Felippe, Felicia and indeed most of the young people in the cities in the *Life Activity Project* could imagine going to the gym and talked about it as either a part or a missing part of their life, mentions of purposive physical activity and specifically 'going to the gym' were absent from the descriptions of young people in the Laverty (2008) study. All 13 participants in the study had experienced homelessness in the two years prior to the interviews and their descriptions of an average week reflected lives on low incomes with few economic, material and familial resources.

For example, Jane and Alison, young women with young children dependent on government welfare payments, did not mention 'going to the gym' at all in their interviews, despite being asked similar questions about health as the young people in the *Life Activity Project*. Both young women were able to recite healthism discourses about getting fit, but neither linked their very regular and extensive walking in an average week to health or fitness outcomes. Instead they talked about walking to the shops or preschool/child care as something they had to do due to limited transport and a lack of access to a car/driving lessons. Walking was constructed as a constraint rather than a purposive physical activity:

> I get up in the morning, go get his bottle, get his food, get a coffee, go to the toilet, change his nappy, feed him, play, watch TV, have breakfast, get dressed . . . This is who I am and I am always here. I spend most of my time with [her partner's] family. I don't drive, I don't go anywhere, I don't see my friends.
>
> (Jane, interview 2005)

> I was actually walking my boy to school this morning, walking up the hill through the baseball park and I thought I'm not as fit as I used to be.
>
> (Jane, interview 2006)

> I go out a lot, usually I look after Kelly, take her out, take her [walk] to the park, go and have lunch, just have some fun; on pay day I go out shopping, get Kelly some new clothes and stuff.
>
> (Alison, interview 2005)

The only young person in the Laverty (2008) study who mentioned going to the gym was Arlie, who used the gym as a site and mechanism for staying off drugs. Arlie had recently exited a rehabilitation programme after years of substance abuse and was very driven to construct a new drug free life. He talked about using inner-city spaces, including the gym, as a tool for self-improvement and as a structure to perform a 'clean' life with others like him:

> A typical week – gee . . . get up spend time on the computer/writing lyrics, the guys are around, . . . usually it is just go to the gym in the afternoon; wake up at nine o'clock. Usually my mates come around and wake me up at nine o'clock and we just dig around until about ten-thirty, go up and eat heaps.
>
> (Arlie, interview 2006)

Conclusion

Jane, Alison and to a certain extent Felicia's accounts raise important issues about the type of physical activity that is available or missing for young people experiencing economic disadvantage and with family commitments in the post-school years. If anything, the commercial gym appeared to reinforce absences and inequalities in physical activity experiences. The commercial gym was structured around the needs of time poor young people with a capacity to pay, rather than those with the least economic resources and physical activity supports within society.

Similarly, the *Life Activity Project* data indicated the gym has taken on new meaning as a mainstream space for self-making, although still recognizing that spatial and social orderings around access and participation continue to occur in sports settings. Through this interplay of space, self and processes of differentiation, young people are participating in or are excluded from constructing related desires around self/body within a neo-liberal context. Such notions support Frost's (2003: 54) suggestions that the market offers not just goods, but 'goods attached to versions of selfhood'. In this way, the gym offers unified notions of 'selves' and participation built around individual improvement, entrepreneurship and a particular type of body that is privileged and promoted in a neo-liberal context. The gym therefore can be defined as the perfect neo-liberal urban space, operating to intensively speed up the self/body modification process, complete with tools and machines for self-intervention, self-surveillance and regulation. Such interventions have a cross-generational dimension (as reflected in Rachel and Maria's accounts), where mothers going to the gym normalized gym behaviours in family life and created a different place from the 'body building gyms' that were written about during the late 1990s and early 2000s by feminists and that still feature in current literature. Such changes demonstrate van Ingen's (2003: 210) understanding of 'space, the body and the re/production of power'.

While young people's engagement with the gym was relatively fluid, the narratives of young people within the *Life Activity Project* (covering a range of school contexts) indicate that young people's school experiences – both positive and negative – had ongoing relevance for how these young people enacted notions of physical activity over time. This included Angela's resistance to past school discourses of a unified version of experiencing physical activity, her new-found engagement with the gym as a source of autonomy through her partner and her constrained, ad hoc access resulting from financial pressures and changing employment. Uncertain work arrangements and changing or limited capacity to pay created variance in some young people's access to the gym. At the same time hanging out at the gym was an important development in young people's use of sport and recreation spaces for broader socializing purposes.

If continuing physical activity throughout the life cycle is a government policy goal and part of the current health agenda, policy and programmes need to be developed around how young people structure everyday routines, demands, influences and drivers for physical activity as part their post-school lives. At the same time more diverse flexible options (commercial and less expensive non-commercial) are also required to expand the range of 'self models' available to individual young people in urban contexts.

References

Beck, U. and Beck-Gernsheim, E. (2002) *Individualization*, London: Sage.
Burrows, L. and Wright, J. (2007) 'Prescribing practices: shaping healthy children in schools', *International Journal of Children's Rights*, 15: 1–16.

Featherstone, M. (1991) 'The body in consumer culture', in M. Featherstone, M. Hepworth and B. Turner (eds) *The Body: social process and cultural theory*, London: Sage.

Frost, L. (2003) 'Doing bodies differently? Gender, youth, appearance and damage', *Journal of Youth Studies*, 6(1): 53–70.

Fusco, C. (2007) '"Healthification" and the promises of urban space: a textual analysis of place, activity, youth (PLAY-ing) in the city', *International Review for the Sociology of Sport*, 42(1): 43–63.

Klein, A. (1993) *Little Big Men: bodybuilding subculture and gender construction*, Albany, New York: University of New York Press.

Laverty, J. (2008) *Finding Social Relevance: young people, wellbeing and regulated support*, Doctoral Thesis, University of Wollongong.

Lowe, M. (1998) *Women of Steel: female bodybuilders and the struggle for self definition*, New York: New York University Press.

Lupton, D. (1997) 'Foucault and the medicalization critique', in A. Petersen and R. Bunton (eds) *Foucault, Health and Medicine*, London and New York: Routledge.

Markula, P. and Pringle, R. (2006) *Foucault, Sport and Exercise: power, knowledge and transforming the self*, London and New York: Routledge.

Monaghan, L. F. (2001) 'Looking good, feeling good: the embodied pleasures of vibrant physicality', *Sociology of Health and Illness*, 23(3): 330–56.

van Ingen, C. (2003) 'Geographies of gender, sexuality and race: reframing the focus on space in sport sociology', *International Review for the Sociology of Sport*, 38(2): 201–16.

Part II
Physical activity and social and cultural location

5 Committed young men and well-balanced young women

Private schooling, physical activity and the classed self

Gabrielle O'Flynn and Jessica Lee

Introduction

Throughout their history, physical education and sport in Australian private schools have been constructed as a means of producing prosperous 'young men' and healthy 'young women'. For example, in the late 1800s, sport in private boys' schools was defined as a process for developing 'the character and values of those who were seen as the future civic leaders' (Jenkins and Sherington 1995: 1). In contrast, the practice of callisthenics and games in private girls' schools was believed to produce healthy and gracious young women fit for motherhood and their lives as wives (Kirk 1998). In these contexts, both gender and social class discourses deeply shaped physical education's and sports' aims and practices on an international scale following imperialist expansion. Thus, while this chapter draws on two Australian schools, the young people's stories may resonate in countries whose education systems reflect similar Euro-centric discourses.

Do such profoundly gendered and classed discourses still echo in Australian private school contexts today? This chapter examines how, and in what ways, such discourses currently operate in these school contexts. It takes social class and gender as the focus for exploring the ways young people from private school contexts make sense of their physical activity participation. The young people, discussed in this chapter, were drawn from two different school contexts or *Life Activity Project* cohorts (see Chapter 1): Bloomsbury private girls' school and Malcos private boys' school. Working within a post-structural framework, we explore the ways social class and gender positions are constituted through historically constructed sets of meanings of physical activity. We examine how meanings of physical activity produce and constitute particular classed and gendered subjects and bodies. Elsewhere, O'Flynn has compared the ways classed discourses are reproduced in government schools as compared to private schools (see, for example, O'Flynn, in press; O'Flynn 2008; O'Flynn and Petersen 2007; Wright and O'Flynn 2007). This chapter compares a private boys' and girls' school to highlight the gendered workings of middle-class discourses as taken up in the lives of the young men and young women from these school contexts.

Physical activity, schooling and the classed self: an historical and theoretical context

Historical examinations of boys' schools in Australia have demonstrated that British public traditions and meanings of sport were taken up by Australian private boys' schools (Brice 1995; Crawford 1986), and occurred similarly in other British colonies. Drawing on a tradition of 'amateurism', competitive team games were seen as a means for building character, moral training and indoctrinating gentlemanly virtues of the affluent 'middle class'. In particular, aggressive team sports were constructed as a means for fostering specifically 'masculine' attributes (Brice 1995) such as being competitive, successful and strong (Dowling Naess 2001; McKay 1991).

The legacy of school sport as a means for developing masculine traits, leadership and moral character is still observable in Australian private boys' schools today. For example, in their study of rugby union players from elite boys' schools, Light and Kirk (2000: 88) describe how the training and playing of rugby union, as a mode of working on the body, developed 'a particular type of physical capital and the construction of a similar, class-specific habitus'. They argue that this class-specific 'habitus' lasts beyond the school and, as described by Courtice (1999), reaches a crescendo in final school assemblies.

During the late 1890s and early 1900s, games and physical education were practised and legitimized differently in girls' schools, compared to boys' schools. What differentiated the practice of physical education were both the imperatives to protect young women's health, and also to maintain particular 'feminine' characteristics. One form of activity taken up in girls' schools included the highly regulatory and systematic *callisthenics*, derived from Swedish gymnastics (Kirk 1998). As well as callisthenics, games were also included in girls' education – however, with careful monitoring. From the early 1900s, competitive games were seen as a means for developing school identity, inculcating moral values, developing responsibility and stimulating mental activity (Kirk 1998). Tensions, however, existed between the development of these characteristics and the 'middle-class', 'gracious', young woman (Crawford 1987).

Given this historical context, in this chapter we are interested in exploring how such historical meanings of sport and physical activity operate in the contemporary lives of young people from private schools. We wonder, 'how are these meanings taken up in the current context to produce classed and gendered subjects?' In asking such a question, we adopt a post-structural perspective of the self, consistent with the broader *Life Activity Project* as outlined in Chapter 1. From this perspective, it is through discourse that particular subject positions are made available to, and resisted by, individuals. Within this framework, class and gender are viewed as being produced through historically and socially constructed sets of meanings. Drawing on Walkerdine *et al.* (2001: 215), class is seen as, 'not something that is simply produced economically. It is performed, marked, written on bodies and minds'. Class is viewed not in relation to wealth or the possession of capital, but as lived and performed – as part of one's sense of self. Following the work of McLeod and Yates, schools are positioned as sites through which social class and gender meanings and identities are reproduced (see, for example, McLeod 2000; Yates 1999). Such work examines the relation between social class and schooling beyond the reproduction of just economic and financial status, pointing to the ways in which schools invite their students to 'become' particular classed and gendered subjects (see also Brown and Macdonald 2008).

Private schools, in the Australian context, desire to produce middle-class citizens who are balanced, well-rounded and successful in many fields (McLeod 2000; O'Flynn and Petersen 2007). Such middle-class citizens could be perceived as leading lives inherently privileged and problem free. However, recent studies have explored the effects of such an unachievable ideal citizen on the lives of young people. Within the UK context, for example, Rich and Evans (2009), Allan (2009) and Evans *et al.* (2004) point to the guilt and constant sense of never being good enough faced by young people, and in particular young women, in striving to 'become' the well-balanced, 'excellent' middle-class subject. A subject Rich and Evans (2009: 6) define as 'no sooner achieved than lost as the standards shifted'. This expectation is also discussed by Wexler (1992) in his ethnographic study of three American schools. For instance, Wexler (1992: 73) describes the teachers, policies and students at Penbroke – an example of a 'middle-class' school – as articulating a 'selfhood' based on striving for success and being 'emotionally self-controlled'.

In relation to physical activity, classed and gendered meanings are viewed as being reproduced (or challenged) through the practices and meanings associated with sport, exercise, health and physical activity. For example, constructions of femininity as weak, less able and passive are traditionally reproduced through sporting and physical activity. Within this context, young women often define the purpose of physical activity in their lives in relation to weight and body shape management (Azzarito 2009; Brabazon 2006; Burns and Gavey 2004; Mutrie and Choi 2000; Oliver 2001; Rich and Evans 2009). In contrast, notions of masculinity as strong, skilled and competitive are reproduced in relation to westernized practices of sport and physical activity. As such, 'it is difficult, particularly for young men, not to construct their identity in relation to physical activity and/or sport, even if it is in rejecting it as part of one's social and cultural life' (Lee *et al.* 2009: 61). High-status masculinity and popularity is often afforded to young men who display sporting prowess and physical fitness, especially in male-dominated sports such as football (Azzarito 2009; Martino 1999; Phoenix and Frosh 2001).

Private school girls talking about physical activity

Bloomsbury Girls' School is a prestigious, independent, religious girls' school located in the metropolitan area of an Australian city. Historically, Bloomsbury has served an affluent 'middle-class' clientele. Bloomsbury students are defined in the school documents as leaders, team-players and adaptive individuals who 'push their own boundaries'. It was through the school that the young women from Bloomsbury accessed most of their physical activities, such as: netball, water polo, dance club, tennis, martial arts, hockey and basketball. The school possessed an extensive range of sporting facilities, including a swimming pool, tennis courts, hockey field and gymnasium. The school also hired trained coaches for many of its interschool sporting teams.

From an analysis of the young women's interview transcripts, three main reasons, or rationales, for participating in physical activity emerged: the material experiences of fun, friendship and teamwork; health and fitness; and, as means of managing a 'busy' and 'balanced' life.

Fun, friendship, and teamwork

Many of the young women talked about physical activity as 'fun'. When asked why they enjoyed physical activity, the young women talked about a range of reasons, including meeting others. For many, school sport provided opportunities to meet new friends and establish good relationships with other students from their school. For these young women, school sport and physical activity was talked about as a means for: making connections with students from different grades; and, becoming a part of the school community. These young women talked about the good feelings from caring, encouraging, and cooperating with others. This is exemplified in Faye's talk about her school dance club participation, in which she took on the role of a teacher:

Int: And um, how do you feel when you are interacting with the other girls?
Faye: Um, I like it. I like the fact, um, like they listen to us, but they still know that we're not being really mean to them, or whatever. Like, it's sort of a respect thing. Like, we respect them, and they respect us. So yeah, it's also, um, like whenever I see them at school they always smile at me, and, in a way, it makes me feel a little bit more confident about myself as well, or just about being around in the whole school community thing.

(Faye, interview 2001)

Some of the young women also talked about enjoying, and deriving pleasure from, the social aspects of sport through being part of a team. For example, in the following quote, Kim talks about valuing the pleasure and enjoyment involved in working 'together as a group' and cooperating:

Int: How do you feel when you play?
Kim: Um, whenever I play a game of water polo I'm happy. It's, it's nothing to do with my performance. It's just – 'I played water polo and that's what I love doing'. I like it. But it depends. It doesn't matter if we have won or lost, like as a team, but whether we have played up to our standard. I mean we all have off games, but when we come together as a group, like we did last year, it's excellent because we play like a team. If we don't play like a team then it's really, like it's worth it, but it's not as fun when you do, when you all cooperate and it's a great feeling. You know, you can win and still all not feel happy, and when you are all together it's excellent.

(Kim, interview 2000)

Interestingly, there is a general absence of talk about winning in the young women's interviews. Instead, a focus is placed on the psychic and corporeal pleasures associated with the challenge of competition. Kim, for example, was one young woman who talked about enjoying being 'pushed to the limit' and the 'rough and tumble' and physicality of water polo.

Physical activity and the healthy body (shape)

When asked why they participate in physical activity, most of the young women mentioned health and fitness. Melinda, for example, said she participated for 'health reasons'; Rachel participated 'just to be healthier; fitter'; and Nat participated because she 'likes the idea of being fit'. For all the young women, physical activity was commonly mentioned as being necessary to one's 'health'. For example, Tomiko said that health is 'just being active. Yeah, I think if you are active like doing sport, I think it's healthy'.

Two particular definitions of fitness were drawn on in the young women's talk about physical activity. The least prevalent notion was one that linked fitness to the physiological capacity of the body. For example, Nat drew on expert knowledge around fitness to talk about going to the gym to improve her endurance and physiological capacities. She said, 'I have no endurance. I'm pretty strong. I'm pretty flexible; muscle endurance isn't too bad; but cardio fitness is down here; just a little bit of work and, hopefully, it will get a bit better' (Interview 2002).

In contrast, the most prevalent notion of fitness found in the young women's talk about physical activity equated fitness to body shape and weight. The equation between exercise, health, body shape and weight is evident in the following quote from Faye:

> You think to yourself, 'I think my stomach is looking a bit bigger'; or you look at your weight and see that you've put on weight, something like that. I think that just generates the idea to me that I'm getting unhealthy, and so that would be my motivation to go to the gym; or go do something to try and make it better; make myself feel better.
>
> (Faye, interview 2002)

Physical activity was constructed as a practice necessary to maintain a 'healthy' energy-in versus energy-out balance. In this sense, a 'healthy-balance' required the young women to constantly monitor their actions in relation to 'eating right' and 'exercising'. As Melinda explains:

> I think that I sort of do because I'm cautious a little bit, like I sort of think, you know, 'if I eat this am I going to be able to use up all the energy that I am getting from it?'. Because if you don't then it sort of gets stored as fat, you know. So I sort of think, 'Oh I'm not going to do much exercise, maybe I shouldn't eat that Macca's burger'.
>
> (Melinda, interview 2000)

Within this construction, physical activity was defined as a purposive activity or exercise, which was articulated by the young women in terms of 'pushing' the body and sweating. Knowing when you have 'pushed' the body, or worked on the body efficiently, was often manifested in terms of feeling pain, and associated by the young women with pleasure. For example, they spoke of the pleasure in feeling sore the day after physical activity as an indicator of the hard work done on the body, and the achievement of some kind of physical change.

Physical activity and the moral imperative of leading a 'good' life

A pervasive theme in the young women's interviews was one that associated physical activity participation with leading a 'healthy' life – which was, in turn, equated with a 'proper' and 'good' way to live. In this sense, physical activity was seen as 'purposeful', not just in relation to improving physical health, but in relation to influencing other areas of an individual's life and contributing to the development of a 'good' and 'fulfilling' lifestyle.

In the young women's talk about physical activity, the terms 'balance' and 'busy' were often drawn on to describe a 'healthy' and 'good' life. As exemplified in Faye's quote as follows, these young women seemed to have no problems in explaining the assumptions linking physical activity to the moral imperative to lead a 'balanced' and 'busy' life:

> [After participating in physical activity] I end up feeling a lot stronger in terms of, like, I don't get sick and you just feel – you just feel a lot healthier, and it also sometimes helps me study a bit; like, if you do a sport in the morning, it helps me to study better during the day. I think it's a good balance. Even though study is important I don't think you should be studying all the time. Yeah, something Emma was saying – she was saying 'It's better to be busy, because it shows that if you are busy and you have a balanced life, then in terms of study you perform better'. Whereas, if you have lots of time to do certain studies you don't perform as well, because you keep thinking that you have got time, and you don't use it wisely, and stuff like that. So it's good to balance it out a bit.
>
> (Faye, interview 2001)

Through the moral imperative of living a 'good' and 'productive' life, physical activity is figured as a practice through which the young women learn to govern their time more efficiently. Such constructions define a 'busy' and 'productive' life as a life that is disciplined, successful and morally correct. In contrast, a life that is not 'busy' is characterized as unsuccessful, incomplete and unfulfilled. This sense of being productive with one's time is exemplified in the following quote from Faye. What is also evident is that for physical activity to be seen as contributing to a productive life, it must be purposeful and useful:

> When you usually go and do more physical fitness, it's more aimed at a self-goal in the end. What you feel is more self-achievement in terms of, like,

you've gained more physically; you've actually dragged yourself out to go to the gym to do something by yourself. Whereas, I think for the hikes, because it's a whole day thing, I end up feeling like I've actually done something useful with my day. Like I haven't gone and watched TV for the whole day, or something. So I think it makes me feel better in that way, in that I'm actually getting out somewhere and doing something instead of staying at home, or something like that.

(Faye, interview 2001)

Those who do not live out the imperative to live a 'good', 'balanced' life, are constructed as not fulfilling their 'duty' to live their life to its fullest. For example, in the following quote, Tomiko talks about herself as being lazy and lacking commitment. For Tomiko, her lack of participation in physical activity could lead to a nonproductive life, and a life in which she cannot point to her achievements:

Int: Why do you think you should [play sport]?

Tomiko: Because I know, like when I do sport, it feels really good. And it would just feel better, like also in my mind too that I've done something, because I'm really lazy, and I always slip into just doing nothing. Like there are days when I think back, and whatever can be done, and I've just been sitting at home all day, like that's me, I do that a lot. So I think that if I could say that I've done sport, I'd just feel good about thinking that I've done that.

(Tomiko, interview 2001)

Private school boys talking about physical activity

Malcos College, an independent boys' school, is located in an inner-city suburb of a major Australian city. The parents of students at the school tended to be in managerial/professional occupations and contributed to a strong 'old boy' tradition and network. The school's website boasts a newly refurbished sports complex, 'one of the best school facilities available', housing a weights room 'considered to be the best in [elite] schools in [the state], if not Australia', basketball courts, gymnastic training area and a rowing fitness room. In addition to the indoor sports complex, the college has a number of tennis courts and fields as well as a 50-metre swimming pool. The college offers a wide range of competitive sports (athletics, Australian Rules football, basketball, cricket, cross-country, gymnastics, mountain bike racing, rowing, rugby, sailing, soccer, swimming, tennis, volleyball, water polo) and strongly recommends that 'each student be involved in at least one physical activity per year'.

Like the young women from Bloomsbury, school provided the young men with the main source of physical activity in the form of school sport. From an analysis of the young men's interviews, three main rationales for participating in physical activity emerged: sport and physical activity as a taken-for-granted part of one's everyday life; sport and physical activity for a fit and capable body; and, physical activity as part of a balanced life.

Sport and physical activity: all in a day's work

The most striking feature of the Malcos young men's talk about physical activity was the 'everydayness' and taken-for-granted opportunities to enjoy sports and leisure time physical activities. Participation in sports unquestioningly played a significant role in each of the young men's lives from an early age within a range of activities including karate, rugby union, rowing, Australian Rules football, soccer, cricket, tennis, basketball and golf. Early introduction to participation came from families and the young men tended to take up activities that their parents or older siblings had played:

> Just the enjoyment really of playing it [basketball]. It's just a good, fun sport. Mainly just the fun of it really, and you know my brother was playing basketball and um, what else, um, and really my family were quite active in tennis as well.
>
> (David, interview 2001)

> Oh well my, my brother played AFL [Australian Football League] and he also played cricket and my best friend was playing AFL too, so I started up with him.
>
> (Darren, interview 1999)

For most of the boys, participation in sport began in the primary school years as part of community clubs. Due to expectations of participation at Malcos, school became the main provider of sport by the secondary years – as David points out in the following extract. The seamless transmission from club sports to school sports demonstrates the unquestioned expectation of sport in these boys' lives:

> *David:*   When I was young I started off sport when I was about oh 6, started playing basketball then and, bit of AFL (Australian football) as well, just you know with some mates outside and stuff like that. Then when I came to Malcos I started playing basketball and tennis when I was also in primary school and when I came to Malcos yeah, I started playing basketball and I was also playing club basketball and club tennis. Then in Grade 9 I started rowing and um, and also, and I was still playing club basketball then and was also playing normal basketball, school sport basketball and in Grade 10 I started playing rugby as well.
>
> *Int:*   Yeah and is there a reason why you dropped club basketball?
>
> *David:*   Mainly the time factor, 'cause you know after school you'd have to, I'd have to race out to [training venue] and play there and train there on Wednesday but um, it just seemed a lot easier just to play it at school.
>
> (David, interview 1999)

The young men were very aware of the school's expectation to participate in sports. As Darren points out, 'Oh pretty much everyone does [sport] 'cause our policy is you must play a sport a term'. Aidan, like Darren, talked about not having a choice in relation to his school sport commitment. Whereas for Darren the imperative lay with the school policy, Aidan talks about his commitment to the team as captain – a commitment that he had to follow through:

Int: So your soccer is pretty important at the moment?
Aidan: Well yeah, I don't really have a choice in that so I've got to do that.
Int: How come you have got to do it?
Aidan: Well I'm captain of soccer here so I can't really pull out or anything. I've sort of made a commitment so I have to follow it through.
Int: So do you feel a bit of pressure because you are captain?
Aidan: Mm, mm.
Int: And so if you weren't captain would you still play?
Aidan: Yeah. If it wasn't in the 1st team though, I probably wouldn't play . . . I don't really like the people in the other teams.

(Aidan, interview 2001)

Seth rates school sport as being 'very high' in the school culture. In the following excerpt, he particularly classifies rugby and rowing as being valued by the school – two very traditional private boys' school sports. According to Seth, these sports were seen by the school as developing 'macho' men. Seth's critique of the school's valuing of particular sports over others highlights its masculinist, sporting culture:

Int: How important do you think sport and other physical activities are inside the school culture?
Seth: Oh very high . . . School places a big importance in sport and it defines you as a person a lot in schools . . . Macho man, if you don't do rugby or rowing then you're a wimp.

(Seth, interview 1999)

Like the taken-for-grantedness of playing sport, competition was also a taken-for-granted part of participating. Due to the interschool sporting rivalry, competition was an inherent part of the young men's participation. Indeed, as explained by Darren in the following extract, the young men were required to 'try out' for a place on school teams so were competing against each other as well as against other elite schools. Such competition made very visible the hierarchy of skilled versus the not-so-skilled students. It also, as discussed by Darren, resulted in prestige and value being placed on particular sports that were highly competitive – such as tennis:

You have to try out for it [school sport], yeah they encourage you to play . . . I chose tennis because it was more select and was harder to get into a team so it was better to play that . . . If you're like bad at sport you sometimes you can get ragged and teased, yeah.

(Darren, interview 1999)

For the young women, competition was defined in terms of teamwork and the pleasures of competing, whereas winning was openly discussed by these young men. The prospect of winning and the reward and recognition that went along with sport was certainly a motivation for them. For example, when asked, 'what keeps you playing soccer at the moment?', Ross answered, 'The fun and the glory when you win'. David also recalls winning second place as a highlight to his rowing season:

David: Highlight of the [rowing] season, most probably coming second at the Head of the River. That was pretty good.
Int: Did you get any awards, anything from school for your performances?
David: Yeah, we got half colours for that . . . Yeah, it's always a motivation.

(David, interview 2001)

Physical activity and the fit, 'capable' body

For the Malcos young men, being healthy and fit allowed them to participate in various daily tasks including sports, Schoolwork, socializing and part-time work. While consideration of body shape featured in some of the young men's talk around physical activity and fitness, it certainly was not a main focus. Instead, fitness was talked about in terms of a 'capable' body. This is exemplified in the following quotes involving the young men defining fitness:

I guess fitness is being able to stand up, sort of aerobic fitness, sort of heart and body condition and I guess food, doing it all on a beep test.

(Harry, interview 2002)

Yeah, um, well I mean being physically able to perform activities for a long time; I don't know, something along those lines. I mean there's different types of fitness obviously, it depends on what you are training for.

(Aiden, interview 2001)

Being able to, I suppose, not having difficulty running for long distances and for long periods of time; um, being able to push myself really, really hard without stopping.

(David, interview 2001)

When asked how you could tell if someone is fit, the theme of having a capable, energized body continued. In contrast to the young women's talk, weight was not the main indicator. As exemplified in Thanh's talk in the following extract, fitness related to having energy:

Int: How would you tell if someone is fit?
Thanh: If they were physically able; um, the first thing that comes to mind is endurance for fitness; to be able to work, um, give out energy for long periods of time.
Int: So why is being fit important?
Thanh: To get yourself through the day, like you don't stress too much and your

body is not too tired like you've just got that rough energy to do everything you need for the day.

(Thanh, interview 2001)

For the young men, fitness was also about the ability to succeed in sports. Thanh, for
example, explained that fitness was important in karate: 'in a small tournament I can
last for the whole tournament, but when I have to do six or seven fights then I'm usually tired if I get through to the finals, so I'm disadvantaged' (Interview 2001).

In contrast to the young women, the young men tended to be fairly satisfied with
their physical appearances. David, for example, was confident with his general
appearance, describing himself as having, 'tanned skin, about 5'11", fairly athletic'.
Thanh described himself as, '[m]oderately tall, athletic, slim . . . Asian'. However,
body shape and weight were not entirely absent from the young men's talk about
physical activity and fitness. For example, Harry recalled: '[y]eah, once I got a bit
fat and I didn't like that so I worked that off pretty quickly. I don't like being fat'.

Physical activity: it's all about moderation and a balanced lifestyle

Similarly to the Bloomsbury young women, the young men from Malcos talked
about physical activity as being important to living a balanced life. For the young
men, it was important to have everything in 'moderation' – as David describes in
his talk about health: 'I'd say [health is] having everything in moderation, like
physical activity and sport and your academic and your social life, all sort of in
moderation . . . I guess social life is pretty good you know, you need to have friends'
(David, interview 2001).

As in the young women's talk, physical activity was constructed as holding the
potential to complement one's academic success. Harry, for example, when talking
about health, describes fitness as helping him 'concentrate more'. His notion of
health encompasses both mental and physical aspects:

> Yeah you've got to have a healthy mind I guess. I think fitness helps with
> schoolwork because you can concentrate more . . . I guess it's not good to have
> high cholesterol, um, I just don't want to be fat. I wouldn't want to be a wreck.
> If you are fit you've got more opportunities to do things in sport.

(Harry, interview 2002)

A balance was talked about in relation to spending time on sport and on schoolwork
– which were both seen as equally important.

> 'Cause like you've got to concentrate on sport and at the same time concentrate
> on your schoolwork 'cause you can't get sidetracked from one or the other . . .
> 'cause if you get sidetracked in sport then you let your team down, if you get
> sidetracked in schoolwork then you'll let yourself down, and your marks.

(Harry, interview 1999)

Discussion

For both the young men and women, school provided a pivotal place of access to physical activities. In comparing their talk, important similarities and differences emerged. Interestingly, the main difference was that the young men were less talkative; or put differently, more extended and descriptive responses came from the young women. Such differences, we argue, are in part tied to: the 'taken-for-granted' nature of sport in the young men's lives; and, the traditionally gendered performance of 'talking' about one's opinions, experiences and lives. That is, the traditional feminine subject is one that is expressive and open – one who is licensed to and experienced with talking about her body, opinions and life.

In comparing the talk of the young men and women, it was not so surprising to find different talk around the body. For the young women an emphasis was placed on body shape, whereas the young men emphasized a 'capable' body (Wright *et al.* 2006). The emphasis placed on body shape by the young women, follows traditional constructions of femininity (Bartky 1988; Bordo 1993). Within such constructions, there is an imperative to participate in physical activity to obtain the ideal feminine body – a body constructed by contemporary consumer culture as youthful, passive and slim. The emphasis the young men placed on a capable and energized body is consistent with traditional constructions of masculinity as strong and dominant. Here, the imperative to participate in physical activity lies with the desire to be more successful – both in sport and in life.

Also not so surprising is the different talk around competition. It seems that the young men were licensed to talk about winning. They openly talked about enjoying winning and valuing the motivation of the rewards tied to winning. In contrast, the notion of competition taken up by the young women revolved around the pleasures of being challenged, striving to do one's best and working in a team. Such notions of competition are mediated by a gendered and classed sporting discourse. More particularly, traditional masculine and feminine 'middle-class' notions of sport are reproduced. Such notions value a feminine subject that can be competitive, but should never strive to win at all cost and a masculine subject that must win and be number one.

Most interesting are the different ways the boys talked about balance compared to the girls. As discussed earlier, the girls generally talked more and they especially talked more about the notion of living a balanced and busy life. They seemed to judge their own lives through this imperative– with guilt and the pressure to manage it all. For the young women, there seems to be no excuses for not investing in being busy, balanced and successful. McLeod (2000: 508) argues, the value placed on being 'balanced', 'busy' and using one's time efficiently is tied with what it means to become a 'successful "middle-class young woman" – accomplished in many fields, with a fully-rounded personality'. For the young men, the notion of balance was present, but not to the same 'lived' intensity of the young women. For the young men, there was an imperative of investing in sport for sport itself – a taken-for-granted part of what all young men do. There was an imperative to be committed to school sport, their team and competition. We see here middle-class, masculine and feminine subjects in the making – capable, committed and competitive young men, and busy and balanced young women.

So, to return to the question posed at the beginning of this chapter: do traditionally gendered and classed sporting discourses still echo in Australian private school contexts today? It seems that, yes, the middle-class imperatives of physical activity and sport reinforced in private schools during the late 1800s and 1900s still resonate today. However, they echo with a 'modern' twist. The ideal, masculine subject of such modern discourse is one who is capable, committed, competitive and manages a well-balanced life. Drawing on the work of Bourdieu, according to Bennett *et al.* (2001), such forms of 'physical capital' and 'dispositions' to health and physical activity have 'higher symbolic value' in contemporary western societies' post-school endeavours. These dispositions hold the potential to 'positively' play out in the broader lives of middle-class, young men. For example, the Malcos young men who finished school made seamless transitions to university study (see Chapter 10). Time previously devoted to organized sports was replaced by a focus on university study (engineering, international business, science) and part-time work. As discussed in Lee *et al.* (2009), the young men also appear to have 'creative networks' allowing them access to support structures and a breadth of opportunities (Florida 2002) particularly for leisure and recreation, as well as a wide set of post-school options in terms of education and employment.

What about the ideal feminine subject of such 'modern' versions of middle-class sporting discourse? Well, such a young woman is capable of managing all aspects of her life – work, health and family. Like her earlier versions, she is gracious, not overly competitive, and she is a team player. Whereas during the early 1900s a future life as a wife and mother was anticipated for the private school girl, contemporary discourses are drawn on to define tertiary education and professional careers as part of the future life of these 'modern' young women. These young women need to manage the imperatives of being career-savvy, busy and balanced, with being 'gracious' and not too competitive.

This middle-class life and subject, according to Walkerdine *et al.* (2001), seems to be privileged and valued in western society. For example, all the young women from Bloomsbury, in the study, left school and entered tertiary studies (see Chapter 10). Such a feminine subject, it could be argued, provided the young women with the discursive resources to construct themselves in a way that allowed them to enter traditionally privileged, educational trajectories in western culture. At the same time, however, this does not mean that the young women from Bloomsbury's lives were problem free. The production of this 'high achieving', 'middle-class' femininity could be perceived as producing highly structured lives, in which there are limited pathways. In addition, the normalized construction of this 'super-girl', 'high-achieving', young woman holds consequences for the production of guilt, self-deprecation and a constant sense of never measuring up – by-products of middle-class subjectivity (see Rich and Evans 2009).

Conclusion

For some time, sociological researchers have acknowledged the relation between the reproduction of social class and gender meanings with physical activity and sport (Cashman 1995). How these meanings are taken up and negotiated by 'modern-day' young people from private schools, however, has not been explored. When talking about the purpose of physical activity in their lives, young people, from private schools, take up historically gendered and middle-classed meanings. These are meanings privileged and promoted by their schooling. In particular, the gendered and middle-classed sporting ideals of committed, capable and competitive young men, and well-balanced, gracious young women have filtered their way into the meaning making process of these young men and young women attending contemporary private schools.

If we take social class to be performed and 'lived', these young people shape themselves in relation to, and are governed by, middle-class imperatives. These imperatives extend beyond the defining of the place of physical activity in their lives. They are also tied to the ways these young people judge their lives and 'selves' to be 'good' and 'worthy'. These 'ideal' lives and 'selves' are gendered. They are also middle-classed. On the one hand, such 'ideal' lives could be defined as being privileged in western society. On the other hand, such lives are also shaped in relation to unwavering, high expectations of success, commitment and high achievement – where there are few options to 'becoming' the capable young man and well balanced, busy young woman.

References

Allan, A. (2009) 'The importance of being a "lady": hyper-femininity and heterosexuality in the private, single-sex primary school', *Gender & Education*, 21(2): 145–58.

Azzarito, L. (2009) 'The panopticon of physical education: pretty, active and ideally white', *Physical Education and Sport Pedagogy*, 14(1): 19–39.

Bartky, S. L. (1988) 'Foucault, femininity, and the modernization of patriarchal power', in I. Diamond and L. Quinby (eds) *Feminism and Foucault: reflections on resistance*, Boston: Northeastern University Press.

Bennett, T., Emmison, M. and Frow, J. (2001) 'Social class and cultural practice in contemporary Australia', in T. Bennett and D. Carter (eds) *Culture in Australia: policies, publics and programs*, Cambridge: Cambridge University Press.

Bordo, S. (1993) *Unbearable Weight*, Berkeley: University of California Press.

Brabazon, T. (2006) 'Fitness is a feminist issue', *Australian Feminist Studies*, 21(49): 65–83.

Brice, I. D. (1995) 'Australian boys' schools and the historical construction of masculinity', in *Orthodoxies and Diversity: collected papers of the Twenty Fourth Annual Conference of the Australia and New Zealand History of Education Society Conference*, Sydney: University of Sydney, 33–42.

Brown, S. and Macdonald, D. (2008) 'Masculinities in physical recreation: the (re)production of masculinist discourses in vocational education', *Sport, Education and Society*, 13(1): 19–37.

Burns, M. and Gavey, N. (2004) '"Healthy weight" at what cost? "Bulimia" and a discourse of weight control', *Journal of Health Psychology*, 9(4): 549–65.

Cashman, R. (1995) *Paradise of Sport: the rise of organised sport in Australia*, Melbourne: Oxford University Press.

Courtice, R. (1999) 'All-male schooling: speech night and the construction of masculinities', in C. Symes and D. Meadmore (eds) *The Extra-ordinary School: parergonality & pedagogy*, New York: Peter Lang.

Crawford, R. (1986) 'Athleticism, gentlemen and empire in Australian public schools: La Adamson and Wesley College, Melbourne', *Sport and Colonialism in 19th Century Australasia, ASSH Studies in Sport History*, 1: 42–64.

—— (1987) 'Moral and manly: girls and games in the prestigious church secondary schools of Melbourne 1901–14', in J. A. Mangan and R. J. Park (eds) *From 'Fair Sex' to Feminism*, London: Frank Cass.

Dowling Naess, F. (2001) 'Narratives about young men and masculinities in organised sport in Norway', *Sport, Education and Society*, 6(2): 125–42.

Evans, J., Rich, E. and Holroyd, R. (2004) 'Disordered eating and disordered schooling: what schools do to middle class girls', *British Journal of Sociology of Education*, 25(2): 123–42.

Florida, R. (2002) *The Rise of the Creative Class and How It's Transforming Work, Leisure, Community and Everyday Life*, New York: Basic Books.

Jenkins, P. and Sherington, G. (1995) 'The construction of citizenship education in Australia: Sir Richard Boyer', paper presented at the Australian Association for Research in Education (AARE) conference, Hobart, 1995, www.aare.edu.au/95pap/jenkp95476 .txt

Kirk, D. (1998) *Schooling Bodies: school practices and public discourse*, London: Leicester University Press.

Lee, J., Macdonald, D. and Wright, J. (2009) 'Young men's physical activity choices: the impact of capital, masculinities, and location', *Journal of Sport & Social Issues*, 33(1): 59–77.

Light, R. and Kirk, D. (2000) 'High school rugby, the body and the reproduction of hegemonic masculinity', *Sport, Education and Society*, 5(2): 162–76.

Martino, W. (1999) '"Cool boys", "party animals", "squids" and "poofters": interrogating the dynamics and politics of adolescent masculinities in school', *British Journal of Sociology of Education*, 20(2): 239–63.

McKay, J. (1991) *No Pain, No Gain? Sport and Australian culture*, Sydney: Prentice Hall.

McLeod, J. (2000) 'Subjectivity and schooling in a longitudinal study of secondary students', *British Journal of Sociology of Education*, 21(4): 201–21.

Mutrie, N. and Choi, P. (2000) 'Is "fit" a feminist issue? Dilemmas for exercise psychology', *Feminism & Psychology*, 10(4): 544–51.

O'Flynn, G. (2008) *Young Women, Health and the Self*, Germany: VDM Verlag Dr. Muller.

—— (in press) 'The business of "bettering" students' lives: physical and health education and the production of social class subjectivities', *Sport, Education & Society*, accepted for publication.

O'Flynn, G. and Petersen, E. B. (2007) 'The "good life" and the "rich portfolio": young women, schooling and neoliberal subjectification', *British Journal of Sociology of Education*, 28(4): 459–72.

Oliver, K. (2001) 'Images of the body from popular culture: engaging adolescent girls in critical inquiry', *Sport, Education & Society*, 6(2): 143–64.

Phoenix, A. and Frosh, S. (2001) 'Positioned by "hegemonic" masculinities: a study of London boys' narratives of identity', *Australian Psychologist*, 36(1): 27–35.

Rich, E. and Evans, J. (2009) 'Now I am nobody, see me for who I am: the paradox of performativity', *Gender & Education*, 21(1): 1–16.

Walkerdine, V., Lucey, H. and Melody, J. (2001) *Growing Up Girls: psychosocial explorations of gender and class*, Hampshire: Palgrave.

Wexler, P. (1992) *Becoming Somebody: towards a social psychology of school*, London: Falmer Press.

Wright, J. and O'Flynn, G. (2007) 'Social class, femininity and school sport', in J. McLeod and A. Allard (eds) *Learning from the Margins: young women, risk and education*, London: Routledge, 82–94.

Wright, J., O'Flynn, G. and Macdonald, D. (2006) 'Being fit and looking healthy: young women's and men's constructions of health and fitness', *Sex Roles: a journal of research*, 54(9–10): 707–16.

Yates, L. (1999) 'Transitions and the Year 7 experience: a report from the 12 to 18 project', *Australian Journal of Education*, 43(1): 24–41.

6 The cultural interface

Theoretical and 'real' spaces for urban Indigenous young people and physical activity

Alison Nelson, Doune Macdonald and Rebecca Abbott

Culture: it's just knowing where you come from.

(Willy, interview 2008)

Introduction

When asked to write a chapter which included the 'cultural location' of physical activity for Indigenous Australian young people, we (as white western women) were cognizant of the dangers of this task without perpetuating a simplification of 'culture' as a static marker. Defining an 'Indigenous cohort' within the *Life Activity Project*, identifies Indigenous people as a discrete group which is problematic in itself. Some of these issues are taken up in the final chapter. However, exploring the physical, social and cultural locations of physical activity in the lives of a group of urban Indigenous young Australians does enable consideration and, where appropriate, emphasis, of intra-group diversity and the ways in which Indigenous young people navigate their multiple, and at times competing, knowledges about physical activity and health.

Indigenous Australians comprise 2.5 per cent of the national population and experience, as a demographically defined group, considerable health, social and economic inequalities (Pink and Allbon 2008). Physical activity has been promoted as one way in which some of the health issues encountered by Indigenous Australians might be addressed (Shilton and Brown 2004). This chapter explores the ways in which Indigenous Australian young people traverse their everyday spaces in order to engage in physical activity. It considers the young people's perceptions of health and physical activity and the impact of their physical, social and cultural contexts on the meanings ascribed to, and their participation in, physical activity. In doing so, we draw on Martin Nakata's (2007) conceptual tool of 'the cultural interface'. Nakata (2007) argues for a more complex understanding of the ways in which Indigenous people's lives are influenced by past traditions but adapt through both continuity and change. He describes this cultural interface as a multi-layered theoretical space, not restricted to cultural specificities, but consisting of both cohesive social practices and contradictions, ambiguities and conflict of meanings: 'It is a space of many shifting and complex intersections between different people with different histories, experiences, languages, agendas, aspirations and responses' (Nakata 2007: 199).

Nakata's (2007) explanation of the cultural interface is consistent with post-structural and post-colonial writings that emphasize the importance of considering: the social, temporal and cultural contexts within which knowledge production occurs (Aitchison 2000; Davies 2004); and, the ways in which colonized individuals (e.g. Canadian Inuit, New Zealand Maori), wherever they may live, might express multiple and hybrid identities (Bhabha 2000). It recognizes the fluid nature of subject positions and that people 'live their lives in a constant movement across different practices that address them in different ways' (Rose 2000: 321). The cultural interface extends these theories to a space where knowledge is not clearly Indigenous or western and where the ambiguities and contradictions of meanings inform what is enabled or constrained in the everyday lives of Indigenous people (Nakata 2007). Nakata asserts that rather than exploring the lives of Indigenous people from western perspectives, it is crucial to give primacy to Indigenous ways of knowing and being, which recognize a 'complex terrain of social and political contest' (p. 197).

Background

There is a continuing disparity in health status between Indigenous and non-Indigenous populations in many of the world's developed countries (Ring and Brown 2003). This gap is narrowing in the United States, Canada and New Zealand, but in Australia the gap in health indicators such as life expectancy continues to widen (Paradies and Cunningham 2002; Ring and Brown 2003). Physical activity is recognized as an important contributor to health for all people (Bull *et al.* 2004; Gruszin and Szuster 2003; Sallis *et al.* 2000) and there has been a recent resurgence in westernized countries of the emphasis placed on physical activity as a means to promote health and well-being (Blair 1989; Booth *et al.* 2006; Salmon *et al.* 2005; Timperio *et al.* 2004).

Among the Indigenous peoples of North America, New Zealand and Australia, there is some research regarding the role physical activity may play in improving physical and psychological health (Coble and Rhodes 2006; Hamlin and Ross 2005; Iwasaki and Bartlett 2006). Most of this literature has attempted to identify determinants, patterns and levels of physical activity engagement of Indigenous people from an epidemiological perspective. Some of these studies have attempted to contextualize data collection instruments for Indigenous populations (for example, see Levesque *et al.* 2004 for their study of Kanien'kehá:ka' children in Canada); but to date, there is little qualitative research to complement the epidemiological studies.

Whilst there are few data available on physical activity levels and practices of young Indigenous Australians, it is perceived that they are less active on average than their non-Indigenous counterparts (Bennett *et al.* 1999). Aboriginal children in the Western Australian Aboriginal Child Health Survey were three times less likely to have exercised strenuously in the previous week, compared to non-Aboriginal children (Blair *et al.* 2005). Physical inactivity and less outdoor playing time and opportunity have been suggested as factors contributing to the higher rates of lifestyle diseases in other Indigenous children (Fontveille *et al.* 1993). However, few studies have sought the perspective of the children themselves.

All young people participate in physical activity within a physical, social and cultural context (Wright *et al.* 2005). Family, socio-economic status and peer influences are known to impact on young people's physical activity participation (Gruszin and Szuster 2003; Macdonald *et al.* 2004; Wright *et al.* 2003; Zeijl *et al.* 2000). However, there is little research about these factors and the broader milieu in which physical activity may occur for urban Indigenous young people. The family context for Indigenous young people is fluid and changing with extended family members moving into households for short or long periods of time (Thompson *et al.* 2000). Like their contemporaries, Indigenous young people are also exposed to current health discourses including the moral obligation to 'eat well and be active'. However, little is known about how they take up or resist these messages.

Indigenous young people in Australia are often positioned as being 'poor' or 'lacking' in such areas as educational attainment, health status and standard of living (Bond 2005; McNaughton 2006; Slater 2008) or, conversely, being superior in sporting ability, often described as 'black magic' (Coram 2007; McNeill 2008). These portrayals are frequently essentializing and patronizing, born of a colonial past that sought to regulate, assimilate and control Indigenous people (Coram 2007; McNeill 2008). For example, McNeill (2008) describes the way in which qualities such as 'peripheral vision' or 'fleet-footedness' are ascribed to Indigenous footballers as innate and likens this to a contemporary version of positioning Indigenous people as the 'noble savage'.

The danger of both these positive and negative representations is that they overlook the diversity and complexity of the lived experiences of Indigenous young people, particularly in an urban context (Nakata 2007; Paradies 2006). They tend towards either reifying the 'innate' ability of Aboriginal sports people or attributing failure in health or education to 'culture' somehow. As Bond (2007: 30) has argued, cultural identity has been used as a tool to predict poor outcomes with 'scant attention given to the meanings held by those who cherish and proclaim such identities'. The result has often been health and physical activity initiatives which have focused on returning to 'traditional ways' invoking a static cultural past which can somehow be captured (Samson and Pretty 2006). However, these approaches are limited in their usefulness for contemporary Indigenous people, particularly in urban contexts. We concur with Nakata (2007: 181) that 'culture in policy as authorized knowledge, as public knowledge, as manufactured knowledge' has become a discourse that enables 'experts to measure, gauge, evaluate and forecast future priorities' in (for the purposes of this argument) physical activity and health education for Indigenous young people. Martin (2006) warns against this kind of 'authorized' knowledge, particularly as it ignores the involvement of Indigenous people and the ways in which they bring their own knowledges and values to their engagement with white, western policies.

Nakata (2007: 142) argues that there is a long history of Torres Strait Islander people remaking traditional practices in response to change and in an attempt to 'reconstruct the meanings attached to our social practices as the context and content of life changes'. For some Indigenous people, this remaking has incorporated sporting celebrations as sites of community cohesion and renewal (Hall 2001). Playing for or with an Aboriginal community has been noted as a source of pride and highly valued by Indigenous people (Kickett-Tucker 1997; Thompson *et al.* 2000). In contrast, exercising alone for individual health has been portrayed as a potentially disconnecting and shameful experience (Thompson *et al.* 2000). The emphasis placed on sport, and particularly football by popular media and football organizations can be a helpful tool for partnering with Indigenous communities in promoting health and physical activity (DinanThompson *et al.* 2008). However, they too can be problematic in focusing on a small subsection of the community and reinforcing an unrealistic expectation of 'black magic'. One might well ask, what happens for young women and those who are not good or interested in football? Does their lack of 'natural' ability, interest or access deem them somehow less authentic as a 'blackfella'?

Consideration of physical place and its meanings is critical in the Australian Aboriginal context given the centrality of land to Indigenous worldviews. Connection with land is inseparable from social and cultural meanings (Martin 2005). Stokowski (2002: 369) notes, 'places are more than simply geographic sites with definitive physical and textual characteristics – places are also fluid, change-able, dynamic contexts of social interaction and memory'. Nairn *et al.* (2003) report that there is a strong social nature to young people's experiences of space and it is important to understand the heterogeneity of children and young people's experiences of their environment and to get their own views.

Drawing on Nakata's (2007) notion of the cultural interface, this chapter aims to explore the meanings of social, cultural and physical locations of physical activity for a group of Indigenous Australians and the ways in which they take up, resist, appropriate and accommodate current discourses around being Aboriginal, active and healthy.

Methods

A qualitative methodology was used following, in many respects, that outlined for the *Life Activity Project* (see Chapter 1). This chapter will present information which cuts across all the methodological tools used in the *Life Activity Project*, but particularly focuses on the young people's drawings, maps and photographs of 'people and places important to them'. During the research process, the researchers and the researched moved between insider and outsider. This was usually the result of the young people's responses to certain questions and happened more frequently when they were interviewed with friends or peers. These fluctuations highlighted their authority in both 'knowing' their everyday lived experiences and being agents in the research process and their choice of information to share or not share (Watson and Scraton 2001).

Drawing on anti-racist methodological understandings, it is acknowledged that 'we cannot break out of the social constraints on our ways of knowing simply by wanting to' (Holland and Ramazanoglu 1994: 133). Throughout the research therefore, reflective accounts of the process were kept and at times in this chapter these are used to demonstrate how the researcher's gaze might be turned on oneself (Hermes 1999).

The information presented in this chapter was gathered from eight girls (pseudonyms used: Kerrey, Jacobi, Tannika, Julie, Jacinta, Soccer Girl, Talia and Sanae) and six boys (Willy, Jayden, Percy, Big W, Damo and Craig) aged 11–13 years old at the start of a three-year study. All students were recruited from an urban school in a major Australian city. An interview was also conducted with a health and physical education teacher and principal in this school. The school catered specifically for Indigenous students from grades Preparatory to 12 and provided transport for its students, which resulted in many students travelling from their local suburb to attend this school. By the end of the study, three girls and three boys remained at this school, although two of the girls had moved to other schools and then returned. Of those who had moved to other schools, one was attending a private school in another Australian city on a sports scholarship, three had moved to a rural area, one had moved interstate and four were attending other schools in the same city. Each young person was interviewed seven times over 2.5 years as they transitioned from primary school (Years 6 and 7 at the first interview) to secondary school (Years 9 and 10 by the final interview) individually, in pairs or small groups as they wished.

Anderson and Jones (2009) argue for the importance of considering the place in which research is conducted as these places can both limit and facilitate the research process and impact on power relationships as well. They argue that 'capturing the diverse intelligences associated with lived space' can be achieved through an 'emplacing methodology' (p. 292) which enables greater insight into everyday practices. For this reason, interviews and focus groups took place in a variety of locations including inside and outside locations within schools, family homes and parks. As discussed elsewhere (Nelson 2007; Nelson and Iwama, in press), we also used 'kawa model' drawings with the young people as an alternative tool for describing what enabled or complicated their ability to be active and healthy.

Home

When analysing the information depicted in the young people's maps and photos it was clear that, as one might expect, home was a central place in the lives of some young people. In contrast to LAP maps drawn by rural young people, their maps consisted of their house and the local street in which they lived, with little else documented apart from local shops (see Figure 6.1).

Soccer Girl, Kerrey and Talia, who all drew maps like this, noted that they were 'not allowed' outside their homes without a family member or friend. 'I have to go with my brothers or my mum. We're not even allowed to go on the road by

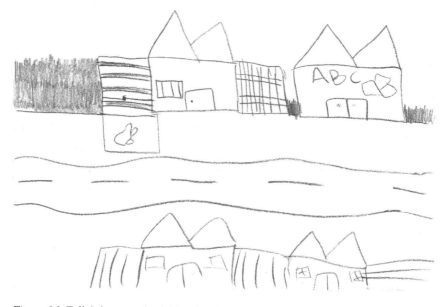

Figure 6.1 Talia's house and neighbourhood

ourselves' (Talia). For Kerrey, this was partly due to a recent burglary at their home: 'we don't go outside that much. Sometimes we're allowed but now that this has happened, we're not allowed outside and we have alarms and all that'. Despite these restrictions, physical activity still took place in backyards with family members, although this too could be restricted by physical size. Kerrey reported that 'we grew up back [in the country] real sporty and that. And moving here there's nowhere to run. You can't ride your bike or anythink'.

Home spaces were used in a diversity of ways to accommodate the family's needs and in ways that contrasted with the researchers' experiences of 'home'. For instance, although some young people had a designated bedroom space, for many there was flexibility and fluidity in the use of different rooms according to needs of the family. This did not appear to disrupt the day-to-day functioning of these young people or their families. For instance, Soccer Girl reported that:

> . . . that garage used to change every weekend! It would be someone's room and then it would be no one's room and then it would be someone else's room. Didn't really matter whose room it was . . . Like I slept in the lounge last night. I sleep anywhere, on the floor, in the lounge room or in each other's rooms. We sleep anywhere.

(Soccer Girl, interview 2008)

Physical activity also included household chores for some young people. For example, Soccer Girl noted that in her spare time, 'I clean . . . I help mum do the washing and all that and just help clean downstairs too'.

Other young people, who mostly mapped their immediate home and street, described how they tended to travel to most places by car. Although they engaged in activities in several disparate locations (e.g. school in one suburb 20 minutes drive from home, touch football matches in a different suburb 25 minutes from home) their homes were deemed to be central. For Talia, Jacinta and Jacobi, homes changed frequently but stability seemed to be provided by the family with whom they lived, rather than geographical location. Although from the researchers' perspective, this frequent moving would potentially be disruptive, the young people often spoke matter-of-factly about moving. Jacobi's account of a house fire ends with a very casual mention of a new home location:

> Nan smelt something and then Nan was like um Nicky what's burning in the kitchen? Nicky looked in the kitchen and there was nothing there and then she seen a bit of smoke coming out of the room and then he opened up the door, pushed it, seen pa, and then I ran in and I had to sling pa, grab pa and had to grab him out and pa just wanted to stay there and put it out . . . he was asleep and then he woke up and said what are you doing here? I'm like there's a fire! And we just grabbed him and then um and then my sisters had to break the window so that the smoke can go out. . . . and yeah that was all that happened and then the fire brigade came and the police and everything. . . . Now we live over at King Street.
>
> (Jacobi, interview 2007)

The stress young people did identify was attached more to conflict with people than geographical relocation. Jacinta lived with her mother and younger sister and had no fixed address, often relying on family or friends for accommodation. This meant sharing space and belongings, which sometimes resulted in stressful outcomes. The woman she had been staying with:

> . . . she came home drunk and started on my mum one night over her baby having a cough and M gave it to her when the baby was already sick before we even came there . . . That lady she stole, she took me and N's two Christmas present TVs.
>
> (Jacinta, interview 2009)

While Jacinta initially contended that she coped with moving around so frequently, by the last interview her comments seemed to reflect a tension with foregrounding the importance of family connections ('They just have this real positive energy about them and they always have a smile on their face and they just make me feel safe'), while acknowledging the desire for her 'own' physical space and the impact of financial disadvantage. 'If you don't have a house then you can't be happy when all you're focusing on is getting a house then how are you going to focus on some happy things?' As Jacinta retold the story of the process of her mum getting paperwork to apply for housing, she illustrates the way in which she negotiated the cultural interface, talking about western systems and Aboriginal knowledge simultaneously:

> Hopefully when she's down in Sydney she'll get her birth certificate. [Be]cause that's where she had to go in the first place, to grab it so at least she was thinking about it when she was down there. M, her name means 'star aurora' that's the same language mum used for my name.
>
> (Jacinta, interview 2009)

Family

Family relationships appeared to have a significant impact on physical activity or sport involvement for some young people. Family influenced choice of sport and the ability to physically and financially access sporting opportunities. Talia reported the family 'culture' in which she grew up:

> We've been around football all the time. That's why I like football. [Be]cause ever since I was born, I was around football. I just watched them [my brothers] all the time and it just looked good to me, like I just wanted to do it. Yeah and they kept saying I was tough enough and I was fast enough so I just tried doing it and I loved it.
>
> (Talia, interview 2007)

The young people also identified family members who actively encouraged their physical activity participation. This was often associated with a moral obligation not to be 'lazy'.

Big W noted that 'my uncle he takes me . . . he always say you gotta be fit and that. [Be]cause he does a lot of walking and he takes me sometimes'. Although most of the young people viewed themselves as active and healthy, they varied in their perceptions of their family's health and fitness. For instance, Tannika noted that she did not think her family members were healthy '[be]cause they smoke and drink and that', whereas Kerrey reported 'we're all runners and we all just take after each other. We all just do running and soccer. We all just love doing, being fit so we can do stuff'. Having a large family also helped to overcome the limitations of space:

> Like I've got a big family and it makes it easier to kind of exercise [be]cause you can never be alone. You won't be alone by yourself if some go. And you can still like muck around and all that.
>
> (Kerrey, interview 2007)

Sport was sometimes seen as a site of resistance when family relationships were strained: '[s]ports . . . it's one thing my mum can't stop me from going. . . . she tried stopping me from doing it [be]cause I was mucking up . . . and she said I wasn't allowed to play sports' (Tannika).

Physical activity was also a site for 'managing' stress or just for thinking:

> Everything happens in my head. No one really knows the real me [be]cause the real me is always in my head and no one can get in there. And so I just keep everything in my mind and tell myself everything going to be OK in my head and that usually gets me through everything, just thinking to myself. I love to just sit there and just think to myself. Do it all the time. Even playing football.
>
> (Jacinta, interview 2009)

Besides home, the young people identified other places that were significant due to the presence of extended family. This included places where they would go camping or go to the beach, or Aboriginal communities in other parts of the state. Talia expressed the importance of connecting with traditional places and the difficulty in articulating their importance to someone else at the cultural interface who didn't share that knowledge: '[a]ll my family's there, that's where I'm from and I lived there when I was little. It just feels safe there when I go there like you just feel like just safe I dunno. . . . I just feel safe' (Talia, interview 2009).

Percy, who asserted that what made his 'life work' was 'family, just family', took most of his photos of family members in an Aboriginal community he had visited while on holidays. However, Tannika foregrounded different knowledge of this place, highlighting the ways in which the young people's experiences informed their perspectives of different spaces:

> We don't like it down in Challing Cross . . . It's an evil place . . . [Be]cause um, every time you go up there people fight on the streets. People swear, people are starting to sniff paint and go off their head. So me and Wanda [her cousin] don't like it down there.
>
> (Tannika, interview 2007)

Jacinta also navigated a complex terrain of family relationships, noting family as both a source of support and of conflict. She illustrated this with a river (her life flow), in which her mum was her 'rock' of support but extended family members were identified as 'eels' who made it difficult for her river (life) to flow well (see Figure 6.2):

> Family can be good at times, sometimes it can be a distraction if your mind's too focused on family. You can't keep going, you can't keep the blood flowing if there's something blocking ya. And family, they can be the worst kind of enemies ever. Who needs enemies when you've got family?
>
> (Jacinta, interview 2009)

The interface between family commitments to sport and the ability to spend time with friends was sometimes challenging to negotiate. For instance, Kerrey noted that she liked having friends sleep over but that this was often difficult: '[be]cause of soccer. Like they can when we've finished soccer . . . but like don't get much time

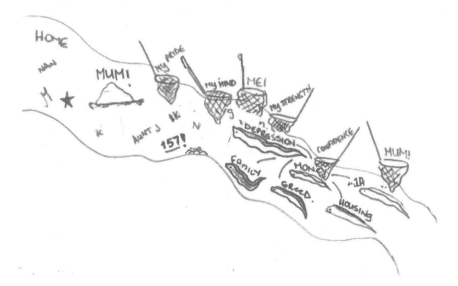

Figure 6.2 Jacinta's 'river of life' (kawa model drawing)

with friends on holidays [be]cause we still have to do athletics so yeah . . . But I like it'.

Community

Some young people drew much more wide-reaching maps of neighbourhoods including places they visited and streets and suburbs in which they wandered. This seemed to correlate with the freedom they had to walk around unsupervised by adults. Jacobi, in particular, seemed to move around not just her suburb but the entire city, either walking or catching public transport. Whilst it was incidental, these accounts show that Jacobi was indeed being very physically active in her area. Her map also illustrates the breadth of physical area she frequented:

> Then we went to the school. It was so mad because I don't know . . . it was just scary and mad at the same time because before we was getting chased and then we was running and all that and then we ran, [be]cause we ran from the Driscoll school, ran all the way to the football field and then we just started running over near the beach area.

(Jacobi, interview 2007)

Some places in the community were seen as enabling or restricting physical activity and sometimes both. The young people identified parks, swimming pools, schools and concrete areas in their neighbourhoods that helped them participate in physical activity. For instance, Jacobi noted 'there's a little alleyway near the shops and we play handball there sometimes'. Parks were sometimes described as meeting places with other young people and places they went with family, which provided the space for games such as football with friends. However, parks were also described as scary places at night and places young people would not go alone. Willy noted that he stayed safe by 'being in the right places'. The social connection was critical in the meanings given to places, sometimes for safety and sometimes because it would be too boring if they went on their own:

> I heard that people get hit over there [at the park]. That there's always fights over there. I wouldn't go there. And I wouldn't go walking around the streets either . . . [be]cause I don't trust anywhere really. [Be]cause there's people out there that kidnap you and there, they can steal you and I don't like walking the streets unless I got someone with me.
>
> (Soccer Girl, interview 2007)

Sometimes community facilities were prohibitive due to the cost involved to access them. For instance, Kerrey noted that they did not access the local pool 'because we got a lot of kids in our family and it costs a lot of money'. Sporting clubs were also seen as enabling or problematizing physical activity participation. For instance, Kerrey and Soccer Girl belonged to the local soccer club and Little Athletics club and spoke of awards nights 'I got medals for shot put, running, and discus. I mainly get them in events like shot put and discus . . . I was very proud of myself'. However, Willy moved from his (predominantly white) football club because 'they don't fix the club up, they just waste it all on beer'. Talia also noted that she had experienced racism when playing sport: '[o]h well like when you're winning or like if you touch someone they'd be like "oh you black dog" stuff like that'. When asked how she responded, her reply indicates the way in which her (Indigenous) coach tried to help her negotiate the interface between sportsmanship and racism: 'I usually say stuff back but my coach just says it's just part of the game'.

Bailey, an Indigenous schoolteacher described football participation in a way which highlighted the cultural interface between Indigenous young people and footy. His comments also illustrate the way in which physical space in the community became sites of cultural celebration:

> . . . In the Indigenous community, there's a lot of kids actually play rugby league. A lot of their cousins, family, all play rugby league so I think it's just a big family thing . . . Touch [football] is another one. A lot of kids play touch because of family and like you know what's out there in the Indigenous community. Like we have once a year we have like an Indigenous carnival and there's a lot of them Indigenous carnivals around.
>
> (Bailey, interview 2008)

Tannika also noted the importance of these sporting festivals as a means to reconnect with family who were geographically spread out. She noted that a local touch football carnival was 'mad' [great] because, 'I saw my cousins from Challing Cross and Windum. 'Cause I haven't seen them for a long time. 'Cause I hardly go back there no more'.

The community was also a place in which the Indigenous young people asserted their cultural and historical knowledges in very visible ways. For example, Jacinta, at age 12, was aware of her political position as an Aboriginal Australian when she joined a protest march in response to another Aboriginal death in custody: '[w]ell Saturday, there was the march for Mulrinji . . . a 32-year-old [Indigenous Australian Man] named Mulrinji . . . he died in police custody . . . And we marched around Queens Park[1] with that'.

Talia's comment highlights the way in which she identifies being 'known' by non-Indigenous people in the global community simply because she is Aboriginal and her struggle to be understood when certain knowledges might be valued over others: '[m]ost countries think like all Aboriginals still live like you know the out-back in the day. They don't really know how we live and um . . . I dunno I think it would give like a new image on Australia'.

School

The physical facilities of the school were identified by Bailey as limiting the oppor-tunities for engagement in physical activity. 'If you've seen our tennis courts, they're so lumpy and bumpy and cracked and like we still use them but I shouldn't be because they're not right' (Bailey, interview 2007). However, several young people noted that the school provided them with formal and informal opportunities for physical activity. Kerrey reported that she compensated for the small size of her backyard by playing in the school grounds: 'we live in the city kinda so it's not that easy to stay fit and so when we come to school we make the most of it, run around, play handball, swim'.

Whilst the school principal acknowledged that the school valued and promoted physical activity and sports opportunities, these were in the context of other social issues that needed to be addressed:

> Well I suppose that's why we don't have you know this pumping PE depart-ment because there's always other like more important things like making sure that you know their health issues are taken care of, you know helping families with finding somewhere to live. Like this year alone I don't know how many families we've had homeless and it's a lot of work trying to get them into a shelter or emergency housing.
>
> (Principal, interview 2008)

Bailey viewed sport as a vehicle for enabling other abilities in his students and like the young people, talked of its stress-relieving potential: '[i]t just helps you with like with skills and stuff like that. . . . I just think sport is a way just to de-stress. . . . I think it's good for life'. He noted that getting and keeping young people engaged in physical activity in high school was challenging at times but that the 'culture' of the school was one that promoted sport: '[w]e push most kids to go and play sport. There's only certain little groups that don't play sport. So I think that's a really good thing about the school, they really put sport out there'. The principal appeared to be motivated to encourage physical activity in part because of the interaction between discourses around the 'obesity problem' and her desire to have a healthy student population: 'I think that it's [physical activity] an important thing for people to do and obesity is becoming an increasing problem'. For one student, the school had taken on additional responsibility to try and assist him to lose weight but the principal felt this had been unsuccessful:

> I feel like we've failed Big W. . . . but I don't know what else to do. I've had nutritionists go out home from the medical centre . . . last year T started a walking club . . . we used to do it before school. You know she got us all pedometers. And the whole reason we did it was for Big W to see if we could get Big W to do it. And we thought if we got a whole lot of people doing it as a before school activity, you know he may not feel self-conscious. But no . . . that failed.
>
> (Principal, interview 2008)

The interplay between physical activity enjoyment and discomfort with bodies and peers sometimes interfered with physical activity engagement in schools:

> [The girls] they don't like going swimming because of the way they look. I don't think there's any girls that wear togs. But also they're all wearing shorts or a shirt. Or something like that . . . It's just in sport like, most of the girls are pretty . . . yeah so just the way they look. They're always coming up to me telling me about their 30-day cycle or whatever like that. And just with some of the girls here I think it's just attitude.
>
> (Bailey, interview 2008)

School also provided a vehicle for interchanges of cultural knowledge. For instance, a dance group operating out of one school enabled the students to perform at other non-Indigenous schools. Kerrey reported her pride in 'showing off' her dances to these other students and receiving their praise:'[t]hey was whistling and that when Jimmy does "shake-a-leg²"'.

However, Willy acknowledged that these types of performance were also sites of negotiation, with some dances performed at his school 'made up' for the purposes of performance. This was in contrast to a dance group he performed in with his father, which was embedded in his family's traditional knowledges. His final comment stresses the importance of maintaining this cultural knowledge as the place from which all other knowledge is navigated:

Willy: They're just made up dances that Anasta College made up

Int: Right. [Be]cause the stuff you do with your dad that's a bit different isn't it?

Willy: Yeah [it is] real . . . Culture I guess, just knowing who you are.

(Willy, interview 2008)

Discussion

It is clear from the young people's narratives that their negotiation of the cultural interface was different for each person based on their own knowledges and experiences. Consistent with Nakata's (2007) description of the cultural interface, they appeared to foreground or background different knowledges in different contexts and in different interviews. For instance, at times they spoke about physical activity in terms of 'mainstream' public health messages of eating well and being active while at other times their physical activity meanings were embedded in possibilities of social and cultural connections (Thompson *et al.* 2000). Participation in physical activity was often an incidental outcome of 'being' with friends or family, rather than the focus of the interaction. At other times physical activity was the vehicle for that connection.

Some young people went so far as to equate their love of football with their identity as an Aboriginal person. Others resisted the notion that being Aboriginal somehow prescribed what sport you played or how good at it you were. There was awareness of the increased likelihood of health issues ascribed to being Aboriginal but the young people maintained that activity and health were their own responsibility and not due to 'race' or 'culture'. Kerrey asserted that, 'you can be anyone to be fit and healthy and active'. Her comment, and that of several others, reflects a resistance to health messages *about* them as Aboriginal people (see also Chapter 12 for responses from young Maori and Pacifika people). The young people's narratives reveal the complexities of their social worlds and the agency and structures within them (Bond 2007; Nakata 2007).

Jacobi did enter into a discourse that reified 'traditional' Indigenous lifestyles (Nakata 2007): 'Aboriginals they was already healthy hey. [Be]cause they used to go out hunting and all that, always used to swim in the lakes and spear fish and all that'. However, Talia's comment earlier about the world's understanding of Aboriginal people suggests: an awareness that she has been discursively positioned; and, an ability to recognize multiple readings about herself in such a way that she was not controlled or defined by these messages (Davies 2004).

Many of the young people identified ways in which their social and cultural connections directly and symbolically created meanings in their physical worlds (Buss 1995, cited in Orellana 1999; Stokowski 2002). The meanings ascribed to these places impacted their engagement in physical activity, both creating and limiting opportunities. At times, social connection (e.g. having a large family) helped to compensate for limitations in physical spaces (e.g. having a small backyard). However, there were often bigger issues at play than liberal messages of 'eat well and be active'. Physical activity and sport were embedded within a social context, which included frequent relocation and issues of housing access. This frequent movement did not appear to prevent physical activity but it did at times impact on well-being. The danger would be to assume (from a white, western perspective) that these issues were all-encompassing, resulting in negative experiences, when it was evident from the young people's narratives that this was not the case. As Martin (2006: 6) notes, 'passion, humour, vitality, knowledge, abilities, creativity, aspirations . . . these are not only to be found in mainstream and "functional" Australia, but also are there within "dysfunctional" Aboriginal communities'.

Physical activity occurred in both private and public spaces. In public places, there was recognition by some young people of entering into a space where culture was being 'performed' (Jackson 2004). For example, public dance performances and touch football carnivals were sites where cultural wealth was on display (Yosso 2005). While there was some resistance to stereotypes of 'blackfellas being good at sport', for some this essentialist notion provided an opportunity to assert, what they appeared to appropriate, as cultural capital. This suggests a reconfiguring of meanings attached to social practices in response to changes in an urban-dwelling context (Nakata 2007) and illustrates the ways in which young people might draw on specific cultural resources in order to make sense of their physical activity participation (Wright *et al.* 2003).

While we do not lay claim to 'truths' about this group of young people in the positivist sense, we borrow from (Lawler 2002) in suggesting there are certain 'truths' in their stories that illustrate the ways in which they negotiate the cultural interface in their everyday lives. It has been important to consider these contradictions and ambiguities (Davies 2004) as they illustrate the ways in which young people lived, experienced and negotiated their everyday lives, and extended beyond the realms that Aboriginal engagement in physical activity is frequently consigned to within public discussions (Bond 2007). The diverse ways in which physical activity was entered into raises questions about the measurement tools with which public health might gather 'evidence' of physical activity with Indigenous young people. The narratives of these young people highlight the dangers of viewing physical activity out of their life's context and suggest we need a range of approaches to intervention strategies that promote participation in physical activity. In doing so we need to come from a strengths-based rather than deficit-focused perspective, where different knowledges are valued.

Notes

1 Queens Park is a large park central to the city where people sometimes gather for public meetings.
2 'Shake-a-leg' is a term used for a particular dance move in Aboriginal dancing.

References

Aitchison, C. (2000) 'Post-structural feminist theories of representing Others: a response to the "crisis" in leisure studies' discourse', *Leisure Studies*, 19(1): 127–44.

Anderson, J. and Jones, K. (2009) 'The difference that place makes to methodology: uncovering the "lived space" of young people's spatial practices', *Children's Geographies*, 7(3): 291–303.

Bennett T., Emmison M. and Frow, J. (1999) *Accounting for Tastes: Australian everyday culture*, Melbourne: Cambridge University Press.

Bhabha, H. (2000) 'Interrogating identity: the post-colonial perogative', in P. du Gay, J. Evans and P. Redman (eds) *Identity: a reader*, Thousand Oaks, CA: Sage Publications.

Blair, E. M., Zubrick, S. and Cox, A. (2005) 'The Western Australian Aboriginal Child Health Survey: findings to date on adolescents', *Medical Journal of Australia*, 183(8): 433–35.

Blair, S., Kohl, H., Paffenbarger, R., Clark, D., Cooper, K. and Gibbons, L. (1989) 'Physical fitness and all-cause mortality. A prospective study of healthy men and women', *Journal of the American Medical Association*, 262: 2395–2401.

Bond, C. (2005) 'A culture of ill-health: public health or Aboriginality?', *Medical Journal of Australia*, 183(1): 39–41.

—— (2007) ' "When you're black, they look at you harder": narrating Aboriginality within public health, Unpublished thesis, School of Population Health, Brisbane: The University of Queensland.

Booth, M., Okely, A., Denney-Wilson, E., Hardy, L., Yang, B. and Dobbins, T. (2006) *NSW Schools Physical Activity and Nutrition Survey (SPANS) 2004: summary report*, Sydney: NSW Department of Health.

Bull, F., Bauman, A., Bellew, B. and Brown, W. (2004) *Getting Active Australia II: an update of evidence on physical activity for health*, Melbourne: National Public Health Partnership.

Coble, J. and Rhodes, R. (2006) 'Physical activity and Native Americans: a review', *American Journal of Preventative Medicine*, 31(1): 36–46.

Coram, S. (2007) 'Race formations (evolutionary hegemony) and the "aping" of the Australian Indigenous athlete', *International Review for the Sociology of Sport*, 42(4): 391–409.

Davies, B. (2004) 'Introduction: post-structuralist lines of flight in Australia', *International Journal of Qualitative Studies in Education*, 17(3):4–9.

Dinan Thompson, M., Sellwood, J. and Carless, F. (2008) 'A kickstart to life: Australian football league as a medium for promoting lifeskills in Cape York Indigenous communities', *Australian Journal of Indigenous Education*, 37: 152–64.

Fontveille, A., Kriska, A., and Ravusin, E. (1993) 'Decreased physical activity in Pima Indians compared with Caucasian children', *International Journal of Obesity*, 17(8): 445–52.

Gruszin, S. and Szuster, F. (2003) 'Nationwide monitoring and surveillance data requirements for health: physical activity', *Working paper series No. 4. Public Health Information Development Unit*, Adelaide: Public Health Information Development Unit for the Commonwealth Department of Health and Ageing.

Hall, L. A. (2001) 'Indigenous Australians and leisure', in I. Patterson and T. Taylor (eds) *Celebrating Inclusion and Diversity in Leisure*, Williamstown, Victoria: HM Leisure Planning Pty Ltd.

Hamlin, M. and Ross, J. (2005) 'Barriers to physical activity in young New Zealanders', *Youth Studies Australia*, 24(1): 31–37.

Hermes, M. (1999) 'Research methods as a situated response: toward a first nations' methodology', in L. Parker, D. Deyhle and S. Villenas (eds) *Race Is – Race Isn't: critical race theory and qualitative studies in education*, Boulder, CO: Westview Press.

Holland, J. and Ramazanoglu, C. (1994) 'Coming to conclusions: power and interpretation in researching young women's sexuality', in M. Maynard and J. Purvis (eds) *Researching Women's Lives from a Feminist Perspective*, London: Taylor & Francis.

Iwasaki, Y. and Bartlett, J. (2006) 'Culturally meaningful leisure as a way of coping with stress among Aboriginal individuals with diabetes', *Journal of Leisure Research*, 38(3): 321–38.

Jackson, A. Y. (2004) 'Performativity identified', *Qualitative Inquiry*, 10(5): 673–90.

Kickett-Tucker, C. (1997) 'Urban Nyoongar children's sense of self in sport', *Studies in Western Australian History*, 18: 81–94.

Lawler, S. (2002) 'Narrative in social research', in T. May (ed.) *Qualitative Research in Action*, London: Sage Publications.

Levesque, L., Cargo, M. and Salsberg, J. (2004) 'Development of the Physical Activity Interactive Recall (PAIR) for Aboriginal children', *International Journal of Behavioural Nutrition and Physical Activity*, 1(8): 8–19.

Macdonald, D., Rodger, S., Ziviani, J., Batch, J. and Jones, J. (2004) 'Physical activity as a dimension of family life for lower primary school children', *Sport, Education and Society*, 9(3): 307–25.

Martin, D. (2006) 'Why the "new direction" in Federal Indigenous affairs policy is as likely to "fail" as the old directions', Centre for Aboriginal Economic Policy Research, Topical issue number {05/2006}. Online. Available HTTP: http://www.anu.edu.au/caepr/events. php#martin (12 July 2009).

Martin, K. (2005) 'Childhood, lifehood and relatedness: Aboriginal ways of being, knowing and doing', in J. Phillips and J. Lampert (eds) *Introductory Indigenous Studies in Education*, Sydney: Pearson Education Australia.

McNaughton, S. (2006) *Effective Literacy Instruction and Culturally and Linguistically Diverse Students: or having the 'tail' wag the dog*, Future Directions in Literacy Conference: Sydney.

McNeill, D. (2008) '"Black magic", nationalism and race in Australian football', *Race & Class*, 49(4): 22–37.

Nairn, K., Panelli, R. and McCormack, J. (2003) 'Destabilizing dualisms: young people's experiences of rural and urban environments', *Childhood*, 10(1): 9–42.

Nakata, M. (2007) *Disciplining the Savages. Savaging the Disciplines*, Canberra: Aboriginal Studies Press.

Nelson, A. (2007) 'Seeing white: a critical exploration of occupational therapy with Indigenous Australian people', *Occupational Therapy International*, 14(4): 237–55.

Nelson, A. and Iwama, M. (in press) 'Culture and occupation centred practice with children and families', in S. Rodger (ed.) *Occupation-Centred Practice with Children*, Brisbane: Wiley-Blackwell.

Orellana, M. F. (1999) 'Space and place in an urban landscape: learning from children's views of their social worlds', *Visual Sociology*, 14(1): 73–89.

Paradies, Y. (2006) 'Beyond black and white: essentialism, hybridity and Indigeneity', *Journal of Sociology*, 42(4): 355–67.

Paradies, Y. and Cunningham, J. (2002) 'Placing Aboriginal and Torres Strait Islander mortality in an international context', *Australian and New Zealand Journal of Public Health*, 26(1): 11–16.

Pink, B. and Allbon, P. (eds) (2008) *The Health and Welfare of Australia's Aboriginal and Torres Strait Islander Peoples*, Canberra: Australian Bureau of Statistics and Australian Institute of Health and Welfare.

Ring, I. and Brown, N. (2003) 'Indigenous by definition, experience or worldview', *British Medical Journal*, 327: 404–5.

Rose, N. (2000) 'Identity, genealogy, history', in P. Du Gay, J. Evans and P. Redman (eds) *Identity: a reader*, Thousand Oaks, CA: Sage Publications.

Sallis, J., Prochaska, J. and Taylor, W. (2000) 'A review of correlates of physical activity of children and adolescents', *Medicine and Science in Sports and Exercise*, 32(5): 963–75.

Salmon, J., Ball, K., Crawford, D., Booth, M., Telford, A., Hume, C., Jolley, D. and Worsley, A. (2005) 'Reducing sedentary behaviour and increasing physical activity among 10-year-old children: overview and process evaluation of the "Switch-Play" intervention', *Health Promotion International*, 20(1): 7–17.

Samson, C. and Pretty, J. (2006) 'Environmental and health benefits of hunting lifestyles and diets for the Innu of Labrador', *Food Policy*, 31(6): 528–53.

Shilton, T. R. and Brown, W. (2004) 'Physical activity among Aboriginal and Torres Strait Islander people and communities', *Journal of Science and Medicine in Sport*, 7(1) (Supplement): 39–42.

Slater, L. (2008) '"Aurukun, we're happy, strong people": Aurukun kids projecting *life* into bad headlines', *borderlands e-journal* 7(2): 1–14. Online. Available HTTP: http://www.borderlands.net.au/vol7no2_2008/slater_aurukun.htm (20 February 2009).

Stokowski, P. (2002) 'Languages of place and discourses of power: constructing new senses of place', *Journal of Leisure Research*, 34(4): 368–82.

Thompson, S. J., Gifford, S. and Thorpe, L. (2000) 'The social and cultural context of risk and prevention: food and physical activity in an urban Aboriginal community', *Health Education and Behavior*, 27(6): 725–43.

Timperio, A., Salmon, J. and Ball, K. (2004) 'Evidence-based strategies to promote physical activity among children, adolescents and young adults: review and update', *Journal of Science and Medicine in Sport*, 7(1) Supplement: 20–29.

Watson, B. and Scraton, S. (2001) 'Confronting Whiteness? Researching the leisure lives of South Asian mothers', *Journal of Gender Studies*, 10(3): 265–77.

Wright, J., Macdonald, D. and Groom, L. (2003) 'Physical activity and young people: beyond participation', *Sport, Education and Society*, 8(1): 17–33.

Wright, J., Macdonald, D., Wyn, J. and Kriflik, L. (2005) 'Becoming somebody: changing priorities and physical activity', *Youth Studies Australia*, 24(1): 16–20.

Yosso, T. J. (2005) 'Whose culture has capital? A critical race theory discussion of community cultural wealth', *Race Ethnicity and Education*, 8(1): 69–91.

Zeijl, E., te Poel, Y., du Bois-Reymond, M., Ravesloot, J. and Meulman, J. (2000) 'The role of parents and peers in the leisure activities of young adolescents', *Journal of Leisure Research*, 32(3): 281–302.

7 Physical activity and Confucianism

Relationships between Hong Kong children and their parents

Amy S. Ha and Bonnie Pang

Introduction

Research in promoting children's health and physical activity is not new, nor is the role of parents in encouraging and supporting physical activity engagement (Burrows 2004; Macdonald *et al.* 2004). However, the majority of studies are based predominantly in western cultures and are conducted from positivistic approaches, producing statistical data (Fredricks and Eccles 2005). In an attempt to address this silence, here we are interested in exploring the subjective meaning of parental influences on young people's physical activity participation within a Chinese cultural environment. By applying Confucianism as the theoretical context, we aim to better understand the social and cultural background of Hong Kong Chinese parents and their children in terms of their relationships to and about physical activity engagement.

This chapter first provides a backdrop of research relating to Hong Kong children's and young people's physical activity patterns before introducing Confucianism as a significant, defining social and cultural phenomenon that shapes how physical activity is located in the lives of young Hong Kong Chinese. The voices of parents and young people in relation to their perceptions and priorities around physical activity were accessed via two qualitative data sets from studies recently conducted in Hong Kong (Ha *et al.* in press; Pang 2008). All interviews were conducted in Cantonese and were transcribed verbatim using back translation method; that is one author translated the results from Chinese to English, while another author did the counter translation to ensure the consistency between the two languages (Brislin 1976). These data are then discussed in terms of how Confucianism may shape physical activity engagement in particular ways, just as the many other socio-cultural markers (e.g. socio-economic status, geographical location, ethnicity) explored in this book.

Participation of Hong Kong young people in physical activity

Currently, Hong Kong enjoys outstanding indicators of health, suggesting that Hong Kong people are healthier than those in most developed countries (Chan 2005). However, because of over-nutrition and/or the lack of adequate exercise, obesity and physical inactivity rates across all age groups are reportedly high (Fu *et al.* 2004; Hui *et al.* 2005; Johns and Ha 1999). The implications of these findings may be that Hong Kong people, regardless of their age, tend to spend less time on exercise and that other matters are more important than pursuing healthy living through physical activity.

Among the social influences on physical activity engagement by children and young people in Hong Kong, school physical education programmes are crucial (Curriculum Development Council 2001, 2002, 2007). With the implementation of the current curriculum guide, the goal of education comprises five components: moral, intelligence, physical, social and aesthetic development. However, the actual implementation and the emphasis schools place on these five components is problematic. At present, only 5 to 8 per cent of the total curriculum is allocated to physical education (Curriculum Development Council 2002, 2007). In both primary and secondary schools, students typically attend two periods of physical education per week, each amounting to less than an hour of actual instruction. During recess or after school periods, students are not encouraged to play or engage in any physical activity because of the emphasis on academic achievements and safety issues (Johns and Dimmock 1999). Physical education is, therefore, not regarded as central to the school's mission (Ha 1996; Johns and Ha 1999; Johns *et al.* 2001). In a study conducted by Johns and Dimmock (1999), school principals were generally interested in physical education to the extent that it produced successful school athletic teams, thereby increasing the school's reputation and helping to maintain school discipline. This instrumental attitude towards physical education in the Hong Kong school curriculum has been criticized for not only resulting in an unbalanced education that restricts children's physical development, but one that also undermines students' health (Ha *et al.* 2004; Johns and Dimmock 1999).

A recent extensive study (boys = 1,065 and girls = 945; aged 9–16) conducted by Ha *et al.* (in press) in Hong Kong reported that, of all participants, 54 per cent of girls and 73 per cent of boys exhibited a positive feeling towards physical education classes and physical activity. When examining the duration of sports participation, 30– 40 per cent of girls and 50– 60 per cent of boys spent an average of three to four hours per week on physical activities, respectively. The perceived factors for not being able to participate in physical activity included 'got other things to do', 'lack of time' and 'lack of skills', regardless of age and gender. Finally, both boys and girls ranked 'I don't have the skills' as their reason for not participating in more exercise. Based on these findings, skill acquisition seems to play an important role in Hong Kong young people's thinking about physical activity.

Another recent study (Pang 2008) focused on how fathers and mothers differed in the expectations and values they placed on young people's physical activity engagement. The survey was completed by 172 boys and 163 girls (*Mean* age = 10.71), along with their fathers (*Number* = 335, *Mean* age = 44.75) and mothers (*Number* = 335, *Mean* age = 40.43). Results suggested that mothers placed higher value on physical activity for boys rather than girls. Further, mothers of boys placed a higher value on physical activity than mothers of girls, but no difference was observed in fathers' valuing of physical activity based upon children's sex. In recent decades, the growing international attention to girls' physical activity has possibly lessened fathers' stereotypic beliefs, while mothers were often less engaged with social shifts outside the home. While these quantitative results may provide initial groundwork in understanding factors that may shape young people's engagement in physical activity in Hong Kong, little is known about how the parents perceive and construct their values, facilitate and encourage the young people, and correspondingly, how young people read their parents' positions.

Confucianism in the lives of Hong Kong Chinese families

Confucianism is a philosophy that has had a marked influence on Chinese families, society and education for over 2,000 years. 'Kong Qiu' (551–479 BCE), also known as Kong Fuzi, is honoured as China's 'First Teacher' and the founder of Confucianism, or 'Ru Jia'. Confucianism includes a set of pragmatic rules for daily living of the Chinese. In relation to this, Hofstede and Bond (1988) indicate that there are four key principles in the teachings of Confucius: the hierarchical relationship among people; the family as a basic unit; 'Jen' or 'Ren' (benevolence) and Li (ritual propriety); and an emphasis on education for the dual goals of economic well-being and educational attainment for family advancement.

Confucianism includes a set of pragmatic rules for daily living. To shape family life experiences in a profound way, a Confucian family may be defined by its unique value system: '[t]hree bonds, five relationships, and filial piety', all of which are considered valuable for interpreting contemporary life. The three bonds, as defined by Tu (1998), are the ruler's authority over the minister, the father's over the son and the husband's over the wife. In other words, parents are required to display love and justice, while sons should show filial piety (the child's submissiveness and obedience to the parent); husbands should show initiative, while wives should show obedience. Parents regard their children as their private property, and they are required to regulate all their time and daily life activities. Based on this bonding, the young and the female are thus in subordinate positions. Females are assumed to play a submissive role by following those in a higher position. For example, a daughter follows her father, a wife follows her husband, and as a mother, she follows her son. The father is regarded as the ultimate decision maker in the family and the mother runs the household and brings up the children. In general, the father is a distant figure, and his display of affection is prohibited towards children, while the mother's role is to love (Slote 1998). Therefore, Confucian societies are often depicted as 'patriarchal, male chauvinistic, and autocratic'.

The hierarchical nature of human relationships can likewise be explained by the 'five relationships', which are based on five basic interactions: ruler/subject, father/son, husband/wife, brother/younger brother and between friends. While the central idea of the 'three bonds' is based on dominance and authoritarianism, the five relationships, on the contrary, reflect mutual trust and virtues among family members. Framing these are the core beliefs that there is no 'me' in isolation from harmonious social and familial networks and that agency is collective and woven into a pattern of mutual obligation.

The Chinese character 'Jen' or 'Ren' is composed of two parts, like a human heart: left – the character for person; and, right – the character for two. Together, they reflect how people relate to each other. In other words, human goodness is never just within the individual because people are always living with others in a community. Living with 'Jen' or 'Ren' begins with the closest relationships. By treating the family with benevolence, a positive atmosphere is set in motion that radiates outward to transform the community, the country and ultimately, the whole world. 'Ritual' in Chinese is 'li', denoting the basic principles of the universe, which underlie all the laws, codes and rules of the natural and human world. On the educative side, 'li' is a behavioural norm that operates through being internalized by the person so that, in effect, it becomes part of his or her entire being. The Confucian rituals are vehicles by which one learns to stand, sit, walk, eat, speak and greet in a way desirable to oneself and pleasing to others. The Confucian six arts, called 'Liu Yi' – ritual, music, archery, charioteering (carriage driving), calligraphy and arithmetic – in a broad sense are all rituals designed to discipline the body and mind so that one can act fittingly in all human situations.

Confucianism dominated the content of traditional Chinese education for centuries. Education has a high status among traditional Chinese values, and children inherit the belief that with the exception of studying, which symbolizes the highest virtue, all other occupations are low in status. In the Confucian tradition, the six arts ('liu yi') became the official learning and the standard for selecting civil servants. An old Chinese saying that goes 'wishing for dragon children' means that parents place all their possible efforts on their own children and hope that one day they would succeed and outperform the rest in their society. This value has been deeply rooted in Chinese families, and parents have a strong desire to see their sons and, to a lesser extent, their daughters succeed in schools, be admitted to a good university and pursue a successful career (Wu and Singh 2004).

In more recent times, in affluent families, sons and daughters are said to receive almost equal support and resources for their education and personal life experiences. Despite the gender segregation, children seek to avoid at all cost the shame that would accompany their parents' loss of face should they not focus on their study and continuously improve. Children's poor academic results imply a lack of parental responsibility. Therefore, 'good parents' have high expectations and supervision of their children's education, which they view as a type of investment. On the other hand, under the Confucian belief, the aim of education is to shape 'the ordinary child' in accordance with 'the ideal child' image (Bai 2005). The Confucian method of being ideal according to the human standard is called 'chung yong', the mean. The mean is the inner reference, the centre of the personality, the alignment standard for self-cultivation, active and positive. Confucius did not dictate what the centre point of interaction should be. 'Chung yong' is the moderating centre between extremes for each person or situation. Wisdom for each situation is found in moderation, the balance between. Therefore, Confucianism, in providing a cultural orientation to education, daily life and well-being, has the potential to shape and explain physical activity engagement.

Hong Kong parents speak about physical activity

Twenty-two parents (10 fathers and 12 mothers), from different socio-economic backgrounds and geographical locations, were interviewed to ascertain their influence on their children's physical activity. In the discussion to follow, the different facets of parental influence are considered: parents' own physical activity engagement; parental engagement in physical activity with their child; facilitation and encouragement; and perception as to the benefits of physical activity. Throughout, we give a Confucian reading of this data.

The majority of the parents participated in physical activities, ranging from once or twice a month to a regular exercise programme of up to thrice a week. The types of exercise included swimming, cycling, jogging, Tai Chi, badminton, social dance, soccer, hiking and tennis. Although some parents reported regular exercise habits, they expressed concern over their participation as well:

> I used to be very active in taking part in exercise when I was young. However, as I am now getting older, I have to protect my tendons and joints to prevent injuries. I think Tai Chi and social dance are rather safe and suit my age and ability. On the other hand, as my working hours are rather long I even have to work over the weekend. Therefore, I will prefer to get more rest or do some sedentary activities at home such as reading the newspaper, watching TV, or spending time with my family.
>
> (Mother of a 14-year-old boy)

According to Confucianism, the emphasis on education and hard work is one way to achieve success in life. With such a root concept in mind, the majority of Chinese parents preferred to work rather than engage in physical activity because they did not want to look unproductive. Furthermore, their reference to health and 'lifestyle' reflected what Confucian analysts would argue as the important sense of harmony and balance in thinking about well-being (Nisbett 2003). One woman spoke of 'protecting her tendons and joints' while others spoke about 'resting', drawing on discourses outside the dominant western imperatives of 'training zones', 'intensities' and 'doses' of physical activity to promote health. These comments are a reminder that the human body, and how it is treated, reflects 'deeply engrained histories and meanings that could not be explained or reduced to biological reasoning' (Warin *et al.* 2008: 104).

Caring for children was also a factor contributing to reduced participation in physical activity. In their role of taking 'good care' of their children, as a marker of quality parenting in Confucianism, fathers placed emphasis on academic achievement. In turn, this undermined the importance of physical activity, both in their own lives and in their children's lives.

> I still play sports but I play less now [than] I usually did in order to spend time with my kids, to instruct them on their homework. As school tests and examinations are conducted quite frequently, I need to help my child to review the test information so as to obtain a good grade.
>
> (Father of a 12-year-old girl)

The family activities reported by parents were usually watching movies and television at night, shopping and dining out. Parents reported that they attempted to organize physical activities with their children on weekends and holidays. In general, fathers played an active and dominant role in deciding family activities with younger children. As the children aged, their father's power relationships with his children shifted to a more passive role, although the children were allowed to go out with friends under the 'regulation' of the parents, notably fathers:

> We sometimes go and play soccer on Sundays, one to two times a month, depending on my son's academic workload or my shift duty. In the summer, we'd go cycling and play other sports more, probably once a week.
>
> (Father of an 11-year-old boy)

> I seldom played with my son and daughter when they grew older. I can't keep up with their pace and exercise intensity. Having said that, I actually enjoy walking and I walk a lot during my daily life. Sometimes, I [go] mall-walking with my daughter and we [chat while] window-shopping.
>
> (Mother of a 15-year-old girl)

With respect to parental encouragement of their children's physical activity participation, a number of parents supported their children's involvement in physical activities. Physical activity was introduced to children because the parents themselves enjoyed it or were proud of their children's sports performance. Being able to excel or develop talent in a chosen physical activity positively influenced parents to encourage their children. Despite the overwhelming Confucianism ideology that sons be accorded a more special status, both fathers and mothers believed they provided equal opportunities for their sons and daughters in sports participation. This contradiction could be explained by the economic resources in the contemporary Hong Kong society, wherein parents were generally able and willing to 'invest' in their children's sports participation, albeit for social and academic outcomes.

> My daughter loves dancing and she has joined dance classes since she was 8. I have always encouraged her to dance because she is good at dancing and always wins trophies in the competitions. I usually watch her performance [with] my husband and I feel very proud of her. Her brother is good at swimming and we allow both of them to continue engaging in sports activities provided that those activities and training will not affect their academic performance negatively.
>
> (Mother of an 11-year-old girl)

When discussing the benefits of children's participation in physical activities, parents referred to three key aspects: reaping the benefits of physical and mental health; enhancing team skills; and, increasing family and social bonds. Several fathers mentioned that sports improved not only their children's health but their social relationships as well:

It is important for my child to do more exercise as it could improve his health. He used to be very shy and timid, and after joining more team sports activities at school, he [became] confident and less resistant to talk to his peers. I am happy to see his growth.

(Father of a 10-year-old boy)

The mothers focused more on personal development such as self-confidence, health and body shape, perhaps in response to Hong Kong's government and media concerns about the body weight of young people. Considering that physical activity and sport are generally regarded as external activities to the home, and that mothers are generally concerned with the home, fathers tended to exert more influence on their children's physical activity as 'head of the family':

I want my son to grow stronger and gain more muscle. A guy should [look] physically fit and healthy. A strong body can help my son gain more confidence and look good. A healthy body can support him to study better and [be] liked by his peers.

(Mother of a 13-year-old boy)

With respect to physical education's place in schooling, the majority of parents regarded it as an important part of the school curriculum but not so much that it deserved any higher priority. Physical education, as with physical activity, was linked closely to their children's academic advancement. The positions held by the parents, regardless of their socio-economic status, reflected a utilitarian view of physical activity and physical education as an investment in health or social networks.

Young people speak about familial influence on their physical activity

Using modified research questions from the *Life Activity Project*, semi-structured interviews were conducted with 12 young people (aged 10–12 years; six males and six females) who held polarized views about physical activity. The young people were part of a larger study across three schools of differing socio-economic status in Hong Kong.

Consistent with the aforementioned study, the young people's perception of physical activity and their participation patterns were primarily related to their fathers' influence. For example, the majority of boys shared their fathers' advanced skills in sports and appreciated their fathers' ability to provide immediate answers to sports-related queries:

My father always talks about his past experiences and outstanding achievements in football. I think soccer is important to me as I want to be as good as he is.

(10-year-old boy)

> For my father, I like it when he teaches me football. He could teach me a lot of different skills.
>
> (12-year-old boy)

The boys' reverence towards their fathers' sporting knowledge and skill resonated throughout the interviews: 'I just talk to my father because he could immediately tell me what I want to know about sport'.

Further, two boys indicated the fact that their mothers were poor at soccer and lacked any kind of knowledge of sports contributed to their lack of interest in sport: 'she just does not know how to play sport', '[my] mother . . . did not teach me how to play soccer as she is really poor at it. I could not imagine how she will look like in playing it'. Mothers were not seen as an active role model in encouraging participation.

'My mother does not talk to me about anything related to sport. There is no time for her to talk with me as she needs to do a lot of housework.'

Even if mothers are being supportive, they are unwelcome, as exemplified by a boy: 'I do not want her to come to the playground. After I play soccer, she becomes very long-winded. She starts to talk with me about studying harder' (10-year-old boy).

In terms of children's perceptions of the place of physical activity in their lives, the majority suggested that parents often talked about physical activity in relation to academic outcomes: '[h]e [father] says sport is useful. He encourages me to join sport activities after school for it will be quite useful when I apply for a secondary school' (boy); and, 'when my mom was small, she used to excel in sport. She thinks that sport is useful when one enters a secondary school' (girl).

These young people were learning that physical activity was not necessarily about fun and enjoyment but rather a tool for self-advancement and as a stepping-stone for a better future. The following quote suggests that some parents were creating pressure for these young people to perform well in physical activity for utilitarian purposes: 'Mum sometimes says if I could swim better, schools may also consider it and let me in. I believe in her' (girl).

Further, the participants spoke of parents placing academic studies high above physical activity participation, advice usually taken up by their children:

> He always says academic studies are the most important concern at my age especially now that I am still small [young]. He says academics will help me develop a strong foundation and by the time I grow older, I can [then] choose whatever I like to do. Well, I am not saying that sport is not useful at all, but I guess my father's right that I should put more focus on my studies, rather than sport training. This is because if I only do well in sport but not in studies, then I would probably experience difficulty in finding a job in the future.
>
> (Girl)

> My mum always talks about academics but not sport. In fact, she threatens to spank me if I fail to study. Therefore I believe I should study rather than doing any sport.
>
> (Boy)

Despite the negative perceptions suggested by the young people, the comments from some of the girls seemed to suggest more encouragement for physical activity from their mothers:

> There are times my mother pays attention to my sport. On one of those occasions, she noticed that I had not engaged in a sport for quite a while; what she then did was to encourage me to go out and do a sport together. She emphasizes that it is good for the health.
>
> > (11-year-old girl)

> My mom is different from my father. She likes to see me doing sport. She believes that sport and academics are equally important. She says that if I am healthy, then I am in the position to do almost anything.
>
> > (12-year-old girl)

The data suggested that boys might be more tightly 'managed' in order to reach high academic achievement, thus getting a better job and being able to take up the responsibility of caring for the family in keeping with Confucian principles. Girls, on the other hand, may be less 'controlled' and given slightly more 'freedom' from their parents in their choice of leisure activities. In contrast, we may see the traditional role of women in Chinese society playing out here where the priority of women is to give birth, preferably to as many children as possible, and thus starting from a young age, parental concerns for their daughters' health is one of the required duties of responsible Chinese parents (Ebrey 1991).

Discussion and conclusion

As a subject of growing interest among academic researchers, physical educators and sports providers, parental influence has emerged as a crucial factor in shaping a child's interest and engagement in physical activity. This is especially significant in a society like Hong Kong, where Confucian beliefs and traditions are deeply embedded in families, giving parents authority in more explicit ways than in many 'western' families. Beyond 'role modelling', where the younger children tend to emulate parents, parental influence was found to encompass support and encouragement, though moderated by priorities for academic achievement. Parents' perspectives suggested that reduced participation in physical activity among children could be traced to their own disinclination towards physical activity. For many, physical activity could project an image of 'unproductiveness', which violates the Confucian emphasis on education and hard work. Meanwhile, at the other end of the spectrum, parents who themselves excelled in or enjoyed certain physical activities were supportive of their children's physical activity involvement, although there was frequently a utilitarian outcome envisaged such as school entry, readiness to learn more 'academic' subjects or the promotion of health.

Furthermore, the father, as head of the family, significantly influenced their child's physical activity participation. The father, who plays a dominant role under the Confucian ideology, could decide on family routines and priorities and therefore dictate their children's exposure to physical activity. In more progressive families, and ones which enjoyed greater economic freedom, both the father and mother tended to agree to provide equal opportunities to children regardless of gender in terms of sports participation.

The children and young people interviewed closely reflected the perspectives expressed by the parents. Young people emphasized the father's influence on their physical activity participation and the passive role that their mothers had with respect to their physical activity engagement, particularly with boys. The young people also spoke of the primacy of their academic achievement in line with the Confucian principle that academic success is coveted.

If Hong Kong wishes to promote more extensive engagement of young people in physical activity, data from the two studies introduced in this chapter suggest that parents, particularly fathers, are important allies in promoting physical activity. Parental education should include information on the intrinsic rewards that children and young people often derive from physical activity and the relationship between physical activity and health, challenging the deeply rooted good parenting priority of children's academic outcomes. Parents could be advised to reconsider an appropriate balance between preparing for their children's future (academic outcomes and prosperity) and living fully in the present.

This synchrony between parents and children/young people is not so typical in western families where children are raised in environments in which individualism is more highly valued (Henderson *et al.* 2007). The discourses of 'lifestyle management' in many western contexts (Giddens 1991), examined in other chapters of this book, position the young person as the author of their trajectory, whose tasks include making responsible decisions to have a 'balanced lifestyle' as they grow in independence. The families in our work drew on different discourses as they spoke about physical activity and familial relationships; one associated with obedience and pre-ordained trajectories.

References

Bai, L. (2005) 'Children at play-a childhood beyond the Confucian shadow', *Childhood*, 12(9): 9–32.

Brislin, R. W. (1976) 'Comparative research methodology: cross-cultural studies', *International Journal of Psychology*, 11(3): 215–29.

Burrows, L. (2004) 'Understanding and investigating cultural perspectives in physical education', in J. Wright, D. Macdonald and L. Burrows (eds) *Critical Inquiry and Problem-solving in Physical Education*, London and New York: Routledge.

Chan, M. (2005) *Diet, Lifestyle and Health: impact of demographic change*, Hong Kong: Civic Exchange.

Curriculum Development Council (2001) *Learning to Learn: life-long learning and whole-person development*, HKSAR: Hong Kong Education and Manpower Bureau.

—— (2002) *Physical Education: key learning area curriculum guide (primary 1–secondary 3)*, HKSAR: Hong Kong Education and Manpower Bureau.

—— (2007) *Physical Education: key learning area physical education curriculum assessment guide*, HKSAR: Hong Kong Examinations and Assessment Authority.

Ebrey, P. B. (1991) *Confucianism and Family Rituals in Imperial China: a social history of writing about rites*, Princeton NJ: Princeton University Press.

Fredricks, J. and Eccles, J. (2005) 'Family socialization, gender, and sport motivation and involvement', *Journal of Sport and Exercise Psychology*, 27: 3–31.

Fu, F. H., Nie, J. and Tong, T. K. (2004) 'An overview of health fitness of Hong Kong children and adults in the past 20 years (1984–2004) – Part 1', *Journal of Exercise Science and Fitness*, 2(1): 8–22.

Giddens, A. (1991) *Modernity and Self Identity*, Stanford, CA: Stanford University Press.

Ha, A. S. (1996) 'A descriptive study of preservice and inservice physical educators' teaching behaviour in Hong Kong', *Education Journal*, 24(2): 45–56.

Ha, A. S., Lee, J., Chan, W. and Sum, R. (2004) 'Teachers' perceptions of in-service teacher training to support curriculum change in physical education: the Hong Kong experience', *Sport, Education and Society*, 9(3): 421–38.

Ha, A.S., Macdonald, D. and Pang, B. (in press) 'Parental perspectives on physical activity in the lives of Hong Kong Chinese children: the interplay of Confucianism and postcolonialism', *Sport, Education and Society*.

Henderson, S., Holland, J., McGrellis, S., Sharp, S. and Thomson, R. (2007) *Inventing Adulthoods: a biological approach to youth transitions*, London: Sage.

Hofstede, G. and Bond, M. (1988) 'The Confucius connection: from cultural roots to economic growth', *Organizational Dynamics*, 16(4): 5–21.

Hui, S. H., Thomas, N. and Tomlinson, B. (2005) 'Relationship between physical activity, fitness, and CHD risk factors in middle-age Chinese', *Journal of Physical Activity and Health*, 2(3): 307–23.

Johns, D. and Dimmock, C. (1999) 'The marginalization of physical education: impoverished curriculum policy and practice in Hong Kong', *Journal of Educational Policy*, 14(4): 363–84.

Johns, D. and Ha, A. S. (1999) 'Home and recess physical activity behaviors of Hong Kong children', *Research Quarterly for Exercise and Sport*, 70(3): 319–23.

Johns, D., Ha, A. S., and Macfarlane, D. J. (2001) 'Raising activity levels: a multidimensional analysis of curriculum change', *Sport, Education and Society*, 6(2): 199–210.

Macdonald, D., Rodger, S., Ziviani, J., Jenkins, D., Batch, J. and Jones, J. (2004) 'Physical activity as a dimension of family life for lower primary school children', *Sport, Education and Society*, 9(3): 307–25.

Nisbett, R. E. (2003) *The geograprahy of thought: how Asians and Westerners think differently . . . and why*, New York: Free Press.

Pang, B. (2008) 'Parental socialization into children's sport value and participation: a Hong Kong's perspective', Unpublished Thesis, The Chinese University of Hong Kong.

Slote, W. H. (1998) 'Psychocultural dynamics within the Confucian family', in W. H. Slote and G. A. DeVos (eds) *Confucianism and the Family*, Albany: SUNY Press.

Tu, W. M. (1998) 'Probing the "three bonds" and "five relationships" in Confucian humanism', in W. H. Slote and G. A. DeVos (eds) *Confucianism and the Family*, Albany: SUNY Press.

Warin, M., Turner, K., Morrie, V. and Davies, M. (2008) 'Bodies, mothers and identities: rethinking obesity and the BMI', *Sociology of Health and Illness*, 30(1): 91–111.

Wu, J. and Singh, M. (2004) 'Wishing for dragon children: ironies and contradictions in China's education reform and the Chinese diaspora's disappointments with Australian education', *The Australian Educational Researcher*, 31(2): 29–44.

8 Being Muslim and being female

Negotiating physical activity and a gendered body

Kelly Knez

Introduction

Through the eyes of many in western societies, it is the body of a Muslim woman (the way she is clothed, the way she is 'read' as being submissive) that makes her appear to be 'different' to non-Muslim women, and thus 'Othered' (Cloud 2004; Droogsma 2007; Dwyer 1999; Macdonald *et al.* 2009). In addition, there are a myriad of assumptions that follow a Muslim woman as she goes about her daily activities adding to the 'imagined' oppression with which she must struggle. Indeed, these assumptions are brought to the foreground when considering the way Muslim women and, with reference to this particular chapter, young Muslim women negotiate and participate in physical activity.

It has been argued by Dwyer (1999) that the clothing of Muslims, and especially the veil, is an overdetermined signifier for Muslim women. This is an important point to consider; as for many in the west (including western feminists) a veiled woman represents not only oppression, but also works to construct a binary opposition between self and Other. Subsequently, when the clothing of a Muslim woman is the focal point of her presumed subjectivity, it works to re-enforce notions of a subjugated, helpless and simplistic Other contrasted against a liberated, self-reliant and complex self. Abu-Lughod argues:

> we need to work against the reductive interpretation of veiling as the quintessential sign of women's unfreedom . . . [and] we must take care not to reduce the diverse situations and attitudes of millions of Muslim women to a single item of clothing.
>
> (Abu-Lughod 2002: 786)

Following this line of thought, it is therefore important that we give serious consideration to the way young Muslim women negotiate physical activity in ways that move beyond the 'western' obsession with veiling and Islam. That is, how are the gendered subjectivities of young Muslim women constructed and contested? What discourses do young Muslim women negotiate, take up and resist? How does the notion of gender (in its various forms) intersect with young Muslim women's physical activity within a 'western' context? This chapter begins to address some of these questions, offering a, perhaps, different perspective of young Muslim women's understanding of and participation in physical activity. In doing so, it is hoped that Abu-Lughod's call to shift beyond reductive interpretations is taken up.

The number of researchers who have been working to explore young Muslim women's participation and engagement in physical activity has been steadily increasing over the past 25 years. Although, much of this research has focused upon physical education (for example: Benn 1996; Dagkas and Benn 2006; Kahan 2003; Koca *et al.* 2009) and sport (for example: Hargreaves 2000; Kay 2006; Palmer 2009; Sfeir 1985; Walseth 2006; Walseth and Fasting 2003). Issues such as clothing requirements and the need for gender segregated areas to facilitate participation have been previously highlighted in much of the aforementioned literature. At the same time authors, such as Benn (1996) and Dagkas and Benn (2006), have also drawn attention to the complex intersections between physical education and Islamic practices/beliefs; and, in the case of Dagkas and Benn (2006), how these intersections differ within and across different geographical locations (Greece and Britain). In addition to this, research conducted by Walseth and Fasting (2003) and Zaman (1997) has focused upon Muslim women's experiences within the broader context of physical activity. Walseth and Fasting (2003), for example, explored the relationship between different interpretations of Islam and how this intersects with participation. They found most of the participants in their study held positive attitudes towards physical activity. However, through using the type of veil worn (nikab, krimar, hijab or none at all) as a marker of Islamic interpretation, differences were found in the types of barriers that existed for the participants, despite positive attitudes to physical activity. Extending upon earlier research, Walseth (2006) used the notion of 'identity work' to examine the intersections between the boundaries of collective ethnic identity and Islamic identity and dominant ideals of femininity. Walseth (2006: 92) reports that although 'competitive sport is not a part of the collective ethnic hegemonic notion of femininity', religious collective identities 'give more space for acting', possibly because Islam is interpreted by individuals differently.

Although the aforementioned literature explores many of the contradictions and possibilities of young Muslim women's participation in sport, physical education and physical activity, it does not tell us about the various discursive resources (including those pertaining to Islam, health, fitness and popular culture), which may shape a young Muslim woman's subjectivity, and consequently, the way she negotiates her participation in physical activity. This chapter, therefore, will explore the various ways in which young Muslim women living in Australia negotiate and normalize gendered discourses within both Islam and popular culture, and, in turn, how this shapes the way(s) the young women understand and engage in physical activity.

Data for this study was collected, in line with other *Life Activity Project* cohorts, primarily through a series of semi-structured interviews undertaken across two years. The young women, aged 14 at the beginning of data collection, attended one of two urban, co-educational, state secondary schools. The schools' curricular and extracurricular programmes required the girls to participate in twice-weekly health and physical education lessons and a weekly, Wednesday afternoon of intra- or inter-school sport. Interviews were conducted individually, or where the participants preferred, in pairs, at school, during lunch times or physical education classes. As will be discussed in the final chapter of this book, it took some time for a trusting relationship to be established but throughout I was poignantly aware that I was working with a group of young women who I had previously considered different, and therefore, Other, to me.

Traditionalism, Islam and gender

The first section of this chapter addresses what is frequently referred to by Western scholars and the media as 'fundamentalism', understood here as 'the strict following of the basic underlying doctrines of any religion or system of thought' (*Oxford English Dictionary* 2005: 367). Fundamentalism will be used interchangeably with traditionalism, which, I argue, is a less 'loaded' term, especially in a post 'September 11' society. Although traditionalist discourses did not overtly shape the subjectivities of all the young women in this study, traditionalism (fundamentalism) is for many 'non-Muslims' the totalizing lens through which all young Muslim women are defined (oppressed, submissive, subservient, etc.), thereby, directly and indirectly, influencing many of the social spaces which all of the young Muslim women in this study inhabited.

There is not one single interpretation of Islam. Indeed, Muslims all over the world vary greatly in their interpretation, approach and commitment to Islam (Saeed 2003; Saikal 2003). Within an Australian context, Saeed (2003) points to four different lines of thought or sub-groups (traditionalists, neo-modernists, neo-revivalists and liberals) regarding the way Muslims interpret classical Islamic law and their approach to Islam within a modern/postmodern world. The ways in which women are positioned within these sub-groups have significant implications for the different meanings attributed to physical activity. *Traditionalists* believe that classical Islam, and its interpretation, is just as relevant for modern times as it was during the times of Mohammad. Traditionalists draw upon classical ideas regarding the place of 'women' in society to argue that women should have a minor role in society. Traditionalists, Saeed (2003) argues, draw upon the discourses of 'separation' between the sexes.

Yuval-Davis provides an analysis of the way women are positioned within 'fundamentalist' discourses:

> The 'proper' behaviour of women is used to signify those who belong to the collectivity and those who do not. Women are also seen as the 'cultural carriers' of the collectivity who transmit it to the future generation, and the 'proper' control of women in terms of marriage and divorce ensures that children who are born to those women are not only biologically but also symbolically within the boundaries of the collectivity.

(Yuval-Davis 1992: 285)

The gendered, 'fundamentalist' discourses surrounding the 'proper' behaviour of women are significant when thinking about the various ways in which some of the young Muslim women spoke about and participated in physical activity. Following is a section taken from an interview with Ranya during our final interview. Ranya's story has been chosen for a number of reasons. First, the way in which she was able to articulate herself has allowed for a large, uninterrupted text to be produced surrounding the topics of traditionalism, women and physical activity. Second, Ranya has been largely represented here because she, in many ways followed more closely the 'traditional' interpretation of Islam than the other participants within this study. Ranya's text as follows illustrates first how she understood what it means to be a 'Muslim woman', and second the gendered discourses and regimes of truth governing this understanding of 'Muslim woman'.

Int: The woman you spoke about that wears the nikab [covers everything below the bridge of the nose the upper cheeks, and sometimes also covers the forehead], what nationality would she be?

Ranya: She's Algerian.

Int: And is that something that is more to do with where you come from rather than your religion.

Ranya: ... who cares where you come from in Islam, as long as you are devoted. Like in Eid yesterday, there were people from all nationalities, it doesn't matter. It just depends on how devoted you are, and what [unclear]. To tell the truth, most Algerians are a bit more religious than a lot of Arabs.

Int: Why is that?

Ranya: The ladies are always wearing long, and one of them, she's really good and everything.

Int: Does the Qur'an say that you have to cover your face as well?

Ranya: No, it doesn't.

Int: So is that something extra?

Ranya: If that's what they want, if they want to cover themselves up more. Why do we cover ourselves up? Because obviously in the Qur'an it says that, because you know, from men's prying eyes ...

Int: And why don't boys control themselves, you said that it is to keep you away from men's prying eyes, why don't men just restrain themselves?

Ranya: Muslim men do, but you see them, it's better that way. We are all human you know?

Int: So why don't men wear head scarfs?

Ranya: Because they are men. Do you see women in Islam going, 'Oh he's handsome'? A woman's body is more attractive. Do you see a men's body and go 'Ohhh'? You don't do it. A woman's body sticks out and gives the whole world a view [laughing]!

Int: [Laughing] Fair point. Okay, so tell me, many people think that Muslim women are oppressed, that they are locked away in their houses, and that their husbands and fathers don't let them do anything and that they are not allowed to play sport, and obviously that is not the case ...

Ranya: For some people, they choose to do that, and they can.

Int: What would you reply to someone who said, 'You can't play sport, you're a Muslim'. If it was a non-Muslim saying it.

Ranya: I'd tell them to shut up and get lost, no . . . some people choose what they want you know? Mum told me that I can play sport as long as I don't get too wild, and that's okay. Some people, they don't want their daughters to play sport; because they care for them, they don't want them to get into trouble, well not trouble, it reveals you more.

Int: So would it depend on what sports you do?

Ranya: Yeah, like swimming, it's not appropriate; I don't think it's appropriate for a Muslim woman, because obviously you are going to reveal your body.

Int: So are Muslim girls allowed to play sport?

Ranya: It depends what their parents think. If they don't want them to, okay, they don't want them to. I think from Grade 10 down, they should. Why not?

Int: What happens when you're older, when you're 18?

Ranya: You're mature, more people will start looking at you, and more men will start looking at you. You have to settle down, you can't just rock around, because you are getting you're . . . I don't know the word in English; you're grown up, full . . .

Int: Mature?

Ranya: No, like . . . like you, you are a full adult you know, in the body and every-thing. Like puberty or something.

Int: You have come of age or something? There might not be a translation . . .

Ranya: Yeah, something like that, and people start looking at you, and a good proper Muslim woman, that's how she is supposed to be, not running around playing sport, she's ready for marriage. In Islam, it is important for you to get married and have children.

(Ranya, interview 2002)

Foucault suggests there is an 'essential link between power relations and their capacity to "produce" the truths we live by' (McHoul and Grace 1993: 58). These 'truths' appear to be natural or 'common sense'. In Ranya's example, the belief that Muslim women cover their bodies is 'common sense'. It is also common sense, or natural that the gaze of men will fall upon women, and that women's bodies are more 'attractive' than men's. The discursive formations that produce these 'truths' regarding the attractiveness of women's bodies are not limited to Islam, as can be seen by my own approval of Ranya's comments. For Ranya, the truth surrounding what it means to be a 'good' Muslim woman has shaped the subject positions avail-able to her, and the way in which she understood her own body.

These 'truths' and subject positions are interesting to consider when thinking about the meaning of physical activity. The meaning of physical activity, and the capacity to access it, is caught up within the production of truth and the mainte-nance of norms. A good Muslim woman does not play sports, nor does she 'run around', in Ranya's view. Physical activity was readily available for Ranya through both a strong physical education programme and inter-school sports competitions, during schooling hours. In many ways, her access to physical activity was not an issue and – as a 'young' Muslim woman, who was in Year 10 at the time of this interview – she mostly chose to participate in physical education classes (with the exception of swimming and dancing) as she did not yet see herself as a 'woman'. What is interesting, however, is the way in which the 'truths' surrounding womanhood have shaped the way in which she makes sense of her body at this point in time, excluding herself from activities that 'reveal' her body such as swimming. The meanings of these 'truths' are in a constant state of flux, changing across time and context, as evident through the way Ranya spoke about what she deemed appropriate at her current age, and what she believes will be appropriate when she is 'mature'. These 'truths' are so institutionalized both within her understanding of Islam and her family that they run far deeper than 'likes' or 'dislikes' for physical activity, or restrictions to do with clothing.

Whilst Ranya had taken up a particular set of discourses surrounding womanhood/femininity and physical activity, Alana positioned herself differently in relation to the meaning of a 'good Muslim woman'. The following section of text follows on from a story Alana was telling about how other young Muslim women disapproved of the way in which she was running around in the park, and wearing 'a little' make-up.

Int: So if someone asked me the following question: 'Kelly, I thought that Muslim girls weren't allowed to play sport?' What would I say to them?

Alana: Well firstly, they can't judge, when you are wearing anything like long, it doesn't mean you are not allowed to move, you are not allowed to have fun. You could be wearing anything, who cares? Like, people [some Muslim women] think 'Oh, they are not allowed to play sports 'cause like, you are moving' but our Prophet said that we should play sport. But these people [some Muslim women] go on as if sport is bad and stuff.

Int: Why is that?

Alana: Because of the way we wear the scarf. They [some Muslim women] go, 'Oh you are running around and wearing the scarf, what's the use of the scarf?', even though it's absolutely normal, [they are] just dickheads you know? Like, even here, [non Muslims], there's a girl; she thinks we're not allowed to do anything. Like . . . we're allowed to do anything, as long as it's part of our religion, we're allowed to play sport; we're allowed to do anything.

(Alana, interview 2004)

Unlike Ranya, and the other Muslim women Alana referred to, Alana challenged those discourses that suggest that a 'good Muslim woman' does not play sport, or do physical activity. Interestingly, Alana was drawing on another set of Islamic discourses, or 'truths' to justify her position claiming that the Prophet (Mohammad) said that Muslims should play sport, and that running around is 'absolutely normal'. This normalizing of physical activity created opportunities for Alana to re-inscribe gendered discourses pertinent to participation in physical activity in different ways to Ranya. For example, with the exception of contact dancing with boys, Alana participated in all types of physical activity at school, including swimming (where she wears long shorts, a long sleeved rash vest and a swimming cap). The meaning of physical activity for Alana differed somewhat from that of Ranya. This difference may be explained by the different 'truths' (discourses), however subtle, that the young women drew on (and performed) in order to understand the relationship between being a Muslim woman and participation in physical activity.

Like Alana, Jasmine also actively negotiated the intersections of gender and Islam; however, she did so in ways that differed from understandings of Islam held by Ranya and Alana (and significantly, her mother). This is exemplified in the following quote:

Int: And how do you feel about dancing?
Jasmine: I actually enjoy dancing but sometimes, in our religion we are not allowed to thingy with the boys, like in bush dancing, you have to swing your partner around, Alana and Ranya, they sit down. I don't tell my Mum, if she finds out she won't let me do it.

       [Interview interrupted]

Int: Yeah, so if your Mum found out that you danced?
Jasmine: She won't let me dance.
Int: But you do anyway?
Jasmine: Yeah, but I don't tell Mum that, and don't tell Ranya though, 'cause they [Ranya and Alana] think that Mum lets me, and if they found out they would probably tell my Mum and then I'd be busted. So I dance anyway, because I enjoy dancing, I enjoy all types of sports.

And later in the same interview . . .

Int: Are there extra responsibilities for a Muslim woman?
Jasmine: No, not really. Nowadays Muslim women have more rights, but back when our Prophet used to live, women didn't have any say, women didn't exist, the only reason they existed is because they are the only species that could breed human children, really. But our Prophet destroyed that, he said that women are allowed to work, they can, yeah, they can converse, they can do shopping. Nowadays, everyone is doing that, but back in that time, when Muslim women were granted, that it was a really big thing.
Int: Some people think that Muslim girls are not allowed to do sport . . .
Jasmine: Yeah, it's mainly because we can't you know, socialize with boys, they think that prevents us from doing sports. It's just a stereotype, and when I'm fasting, they [people at school] go, 'Oh are you allowed to watch

TV when you are fasting?', I mean what has that got to do with anything? They ask 'Would you get whipped if you talk to a boy?' I'm like 'Where did you get that from?' There are just things, because we can't socialize with boys, wear mini skirts, go out and play netball because that's the standard uniform for it, they think that prevents us from doing physical activity.

Int: And does it?

Jasmine: No.

Int: Does Islam provide any barriers to you doing physical activity?

Jasmine: No, I don't think there are any barriers.

(Jasmine, interview 2004)

Whilst the gendered discourses associated with Islam and what it means to be a young Muslim woman are significant, the earlier data from Ranya, Alana and Jasmine demonstrates the complexity of this relationship. Furthermore, the talk of these three young women acts as a reminder of the different ways in which young Muslim women can negotiate their own understandings of Islam, what it means to be a young Muslim women and how this shapes the way they make meaning of physical activity. The complex nature of this intersection is further demonstrated when we consider that these three young women are friends, that they belong to the same Muslim community and that their families have regular contact with each other. Despite the young women inhabiting similar social spaces, there has been opportunity for each of them to shape their own subjectivities in different ways, however subtle.

Popular culture

Whilst the earlier data provides a powerful example of difference between the participants, this section will demonstrate the significance of normalization with a specific focus upon how the young women constitute themselves through normalized feminine discourses from popular culture. Like the young women in Oliver's (1999) study, the young Muslim women were acutely aware of their bodies in relation to gendered images found within popular culture, which are portrayed and represented as being 'normal'. The various examples of data within this section have been taken from the magazine interview transcripts. The two magazines used to facilitate discussion were *Women in Sport* and *Chick*. Oliver (1999), in her paper *Adolescent girls' body-narratives: Learning to desire and create a "fashionable" image*, describes how the adolescent girls in her study constructed the meanings of their bodies through fashion. She found that images were a powerful source of knowing for subjects, not only were they 'using images as an interpretative frame for learning about their worlds, their selves, and specifically their bodies, they were often accepting the visual images they saw at "face value"' (Oliver 1999: 243). Through their consumption of fashion images and ideas, the girls in her study were learning to create a desirable image, which they associated with being normal (perfect look, hair, body, clothes, etc.). All of the young women in my study regularly read magazines whose intended audience was female. Although the participants' access to magazines varied from reading their mothers' magazines (*Woman's Day*, *New Idea*, *Woman's Weekly*, etc.), to either their own or friends' copies (*Dolly*, *Marie Claire* and *Cosmopolitan*), the pictures within the magazines provide stereotypical images of what a female body 'should' look like.

All 11 young women in describing/evaluating their own bodies drew on discourses from popular culture and contemporary western culture that constituted a 'normal' female body, as one which was neither fat, nor skinny, and was especially not too muscly. The participants had a very clear understanding of what a young woman's body should look like and that it should in no way resemble that of a man's body. This is particularly evident in comments made by Maria, Jasmine and Zeena who claimed that muscles looked 'really bad' on women, and that girls who worked out too much and had a 'six pack' looked 'disgusting'. Additionally, Kameela spoke of following an abdominal exercise regime outlined in a magazine, not intending to gain muscles but with the aim of loosing the 'unnatural fat' on her body. Similarly, Jasmine stated that girls can exercise, but not 'too much', and that girls should not be weightlifters. The young women constructed their own understanding of gender and what a young woman's body should look like, using 'binary logic': 'which constitutes the world in hierarchical ways through its privileging of one term or category within the binary and depriving the opposite term of meaning in its own right' (Davies 2000: 107). That is, to successfully constitute themselves as female, they were only too aware of the 'work' they need to do in order to maintain the gender order of which they are a part. In this instance, it was to ensure a body which was clearly 'female', slim, but not too muscly. Indeed, this served to reenforce the strong gendered discourses of fundamentalism, further narrowing the way some of the participants were able to understand themselves as female.

Heteronormativity and marriage

Whilst the young Muslim women shared with their non-Muslim peers many similarities, one of the striking differences was the way some of the young Muslim women spoke about marriage. The talk of the participants extended well beyond passing comments such as 'oh, one day I'll get married', or 'when I'm married . . .'. How three of the young women, in particular, spoke about their own future marriages, and their mothers' investment/interest in this institution, sheds significant light on why the participants dress modestly, and are under constant surveillance by themselves and their families to successfully constitute themselves within the female gender category. Whilst all of the participants spoke about marriage, the four women quoted in this section spoke in considerably more detail about marriage than the other participants.

Following is a section of data taken from the health and fitness interview with Jasmine. It illustrates the significance of both normalized feminine discourses, and those relating to heteronormativity and marriage.

Int: Is there, are there any expectations placed on you because you are a Muslim women, in terms of when you grow up?

Jasmine:	My parents expect me to marry. I'm not so hot about that.
Int:	Why do they expect you to marry?
Jasmine:	I don't know.
Int:	Is it a cultural thing?
Jasmine:	She just wants me to marry, I think she just wants grandchildren [laughing].
Int:	Don't worry, my Mum wants grandchildren too, I told her she can wait [laughing].
Jasmine:	[Laughing].
Int:	So ...
Jasmine:	I think that's all, and she wants me to be a good, 'cause in our religion it is absolutely forbidden to bed anyone until you marry, you have to stay as a virgin and stuff. She doesn't want me to grow up and be one of those funk girls, you know pierced everywhere, go around drinking alcohol, beer, a whore or anything. She goes, 'I want you to be a proper girl, that's all, and have a good job'.

(Jasmine, interview 2004)

The earlier exchange indicates how normalizing discourses, which associate maturity with marriage(ability), limit the ways Jasmine is able to constitute herself as 'female'. For example, how her mother's injunction to be a 'good' and 'proper girl' excludes her from being 'funky', having body piercing, drinking alcohol or expressing her sexuality. The emphasis on marriage(ability) reinforces the investment Jasmine must make in ensuring she not only constitutes herself within the female category, but that she also constitutes herself as a 'proper girl'.

Jasmine's comments also remind us, however, that where power exists, so too do opportunities for resistance. Although the subject is socially constructed, she is also capable, to a degree, of reflecting upon the discursive resources available, and choosing to take these up or resist them (Weedon 1989). In the earlier example, Jasmine is beginning to resist her mother's expectation of her marrying. This is further supported in statements made by Jasmine during other interviews in which she expresses her desire to follow her own path, and make her own choices rather than following the expectations of her parents. On the other hand, whilst the earlier text suggests Jasmine's capabilities of resisting and/or agency, her prior comments regarding girls exercising (but not 'too' much) remind us of the persuasiveness of dominant feminine discourses and the privileging of stability (and normalization) within gender categories. Whilst she may be able to resist her parents' expectations of marriage, it is still difficult for her to constitute herself as anything but a 'normal' female, the same 'normal' female that her mother would prefer her to be. Following are further examples from interviews with Zeena, Alana and Ranya of the ways both feminine discourses were taken up by the young women.

Int:	And what does your Mum think about you using the exercise bike.
Zeena:	She says, 'You don't need to exercise, just diet, if you want to go skinny', but she goes 'You're totally fine at the moment'. Like right now, 'cause

my Indian clothes won't fit me, she's like, 'Your hips are getting bigger', and I'm like, 'What do you mean my hips are getting bigger, I'm a girl, what do you expect?' You know?

Int: Yeah.

Zeena: Yeah, but she wants me to be skinny, she doesn't want me to go fat.

Int: Why does she want you to be skinny?

Zeena: 'Cause she's fat.

Int: Do you think that's the only reason why, because . . .

Zeena: Oh I don't know, she just wants me to be healthy, you know, because I'm going to get mar-r-ied, and if I'm fat, then no one will want to mar-ry me.

Int: And how does that make you feel?

Zeena: But I've got seven marriage proposals anyway.

Int: How many have you had?

Zeena: Seven, already, so I don't know what she's worried about. I'm like 'It doesn't matter, geez'.

(Zeena, interview 2002)

Alana and Ranya:

Int: Why is your Mum, why are your Mums concerned about your bodies?

Alana: About marriage, you know . . .

Ranya: You know, they think, 'What are we going to do with you when you grow up? No one will want you'.

Alana: And they say you will grow fat, and you will be ashamed of going outside. And when you're female, and you get ashamed because your clothes don't fit you properly and everybody looks at you just because you are fat, and everything. That's what they [mothers] are concerned about, you know.

(Alana and Ranya, interview 2003)

Marriage is, for these young women, an important component of their Islamic culture. Alana, Ranya and Zeena have accepted the way in which dominant feminine discourses position them as young Muslim women. In order to optimize this position (through securing an appropriate husband), these three young women worked hard to constitute themselves as 'normal' females with the 'right' body shape. Whilst this could be viewed as an example of the subordination of women, McNay argues that there is a significant 'pay off' for some women taking up such discourses:

> The notion of investment helps to explain the kinds of 'reward' women obtain from placing themselves in positions which are commonly regarded as subordinate. Thus, quoting a study by Angela McRobbie on adolescent, working-class girls and their ambition to 'attract and keep a man', Holloway argues that commonly accepted practices of femininity take it for granted that there is status and power attached to attracting and possessing men. Thus, what is often perceived as the subordination of women to male demands and desires, is not

necessarily experienced as such by those women, but rather as an expression of their power.

(McNay 1992: 82)

For these young women, and indeed their parents, marriage as an expression of power, can be likened to Foucault's notion of power as a 'productive' force (Foucault 1980). In the earlier examples, the normalizing power of heterosexuality, which is publicly demonstrated through marriage, provides significant 'pay-offs' which may include social status and acceptance (as being a 'normal' Muslim/woman) and increased financial security. However, whilst power can produce new capabilities, and enable change, normalized power is difficult to resist. The reward for successfully constituting oneself as a 'normal' heterosexual female and, in the case of the aforementioned participants, a 'good' and/or 'proper' female is unquestionably significant. However, it comes at the expense of different and varied subject positions (such as different ways of being and living as a young Muslim woman) through which the participants can understand their bodies, and, indeed, their participation in physical activity.

Conclusion

This chapter has sought to explore the notion of a gendered body and how this intersects with physical activity through the lived experiences of the young Muslim women who participated in this research. In particular, it has attempted to understand the gendered experiences of young Muslim women, and their relationship to physical activity, without a reductive focus on clothing. As Davies (2000: 62) states, 'we are constituted as gendered through complex metaphors and storylines that constitute (and through which we constitute) ourselves as embodied and desiring beings'. Whilst the subjectivities of the young women were shaped by dominant feminine discourses from both Islam and popular culture, the ways in which these discourses were negotiated, taken up and resisted varied. These variations were dependant upon the young women's access to multiple ways of 'knowing' and 'being', which changed according to the subject positions they were able to take up. The meaning and place of physical activity in the lives of young Muslim women in this study was shaped by the various 'truths' associated with what it means to be a 'normal woman', and how these intersected with discourses of religion, popular culture and heteronormativity.

Whilst variations in embodied subjectivities can be explained by the young women having access to different subject positions, there appears to be a significant pay-off for taking up those subject positions which are deemed to be 'normal'. This is particularly evident for these young women when considering the way heteronormative discourses were first embodied through constituting themselves as female, and thus different to men, and second the way this was publicly displayed through marriage. The young women presented within this chapter had a very clear understanding of what their bodies should look like. This is further reinforced by the expectation (from their mothers) that they will get married.

Giving consideration to the different and complex ways in which young Muslim women constitute themselves as female allows a shift away from reductive and 'western' obsessions with Muslim women's clothing and, in particular, the veil. For the young women in this study, gender was indeed significant in both shaping their access to, and participation in, physical activity. This was especially so when the young women 'knew' how they needed to look (from both a religious and gendered perspective), and the types of physical activity they would participate in as a result.

References

Abu-Lughod, L. (2002) 'Do Muslim women really need saving? Anthropological reflections on cultural relativism and its Others', *American Anthropologist*, 104(3): 783–90.

Benn, T. (1996) 'Muslim women and physical education in initial teacher training', *Sport, Education and Society*, 1(1): 5–21.

Cloud, D. L. (2004) 'To veil the threat of terror: Afghan women and the clash of civilizations in the imaginary of the U.S. war on terrorism', *Quarterly Journal of Speech*, 90(3): 285–306.

Dagkas, S. and Benn, T. (2006) 'Young Muslim women's experiences of Islam and physical education in Greece and Britain: a comparative study', *Sport, Education and Society*, 11(1): 21–88.

Davies, B. (2000) *A Body of Writing 1990–1999*, Walnut Creek, CA: Altamira Press.

Droogsma, R. A. (2007) 'Redefining Hijab: American Muslim women's standpoints of veiling', *Journal of Applied Communication Research*, 35(3): 294–319.

Dwyer, C. (1999) 'Veiled meanings: young British Muslim women and the negotiation of difference', *Gender, Place and Society*, 6(1): 5–26.

Foucault, M. (1980) *Power/Knowledge: selected interviews and other writings*, Brighton: The Harvester Press.

Hargreaves, J. (2000) *Heroines of Sport: the politics of difference and identity*, New York: Routledge.

Kahan, D. (2003) 'Islam and physical activity: implications for American sport and physical education', *Journal of Physical Education, Recreation and Dance*, 74(3): 48–54.

Kay, T. (2006) 'Daughters of Islam: family influences on Muslim young women's participation in sport', *International Review for the Sociology of Sport*, 41(3): 357–73.

Koca, C., Atencio, M. and Demirhan, G. (2009) 'The place and meaning of the field of PE in Turkish young people's lives: a study using Bourdieu's conceptual tools', *Sport, Education and Society*, 14(1): 55–75.

Macdonald, D., Abbott, R., Knez, K. and Nelson, A. (2009) 'Taking exercise: cultural diversity and physically active lifestyles', *Sport, Education and Society*, 14(1): 1–20.

McHoul, A. and Grace, W. (1993) *A Foucault Primer: discourse, power and the subject*, Carlton: Melbourne University Press.

McNay, L. (1992) *Foucault and Feminism: power, gender and the self*, Cambridge: Polity Press.

Oliver, K. (1999) 'Adolescent girl's body-narratives: Learning to desire and create a "fashionable" image' *Teacher College Record*, 10(2): 220–246.

Oxford English Dictionary (2005) Oxford and New York: Oxford University Press.

Palmer, C. (2009) 'Soccer and the politics of identity for young Muslim refugee women in South Australia', *Soccer and Society*, 10(1): 27–38.

Saeed, A. (2003) *Islam in Australia*, Crows Nest, NSW: Allen & Unwin.

Saikal, A. (2003) *Islam and the West: conflict or cooperation?*, New York: Palgrave Macmillan.

Sfeir, L. (1985) 'The status of Muslim women in sport: conflict between cultural tradition and modernization', *International Review for the Sociology of Sport*, 20(4): 283–305.

Walseth, K. (2006) 'Young Muslim women and sport: the impact of identity work', *Leisure Studies*, 25(1): 75–94.

Walseth, K. and Fasting, K. (2003) 'Islam's view on physical activity and sport: Egyptian women interpreting Islam', *International Review for the Sociology of Sport*, 38(1): 45–60.

Weedon, C. (1989) *Feminist Practice and Post-Structuralist Theory*, Oxford: Blackwell Publishing.

Yuval-Davis, N. (1992) 'Fundamentalism, multiculturalism and women', in J. Donald and A. Rattansi (eds) *Race, Culture and Difference*, London: Sage with the Open University.

Zaman, H. (1997) 'Islam, well-being and physical activity: perceptions of Muslim young women', in G. Clark and B. Humberstone (eds) *Researching Women and Sport*, London: Macmillan Press.

Part III

Physical activity and the constitution of healthy, fit bodies

9 Anxieties and aspirations

The making of active, informed citizens

Doune Macdonald, Jan Wright and Rebecca Abbott

In writing *The Code of Health and Longevity* in 1818, Sir John Sinclair hoped that with the provision:

> of the facts and observations, which are *most essential* for the preservation of health, . . . that it will now be in the power of every considerable person, to ascertain what rules are suited to his particular situation, and to adopt those which are likely to be most efficacious.
>
> (Sinclair 1818: 13)

Motivating Sir John's tome nearly 200 years ago was his concern that 'people seldom attend to their health till it be too late' (p. 12) and that 'the attainment of longevity, if accompanied with good health, is not only an important consideration to the individual, but also to the community to which he belongs' (p. 12).

Since that time, persuading citizens to take responsibility for their health and well-being has become a preoccupation of governments in most Western democracies. These government are said to be largely driven by neo-liberalism, with its emphasis on cost-containment, shrinking of the state and a freeing of the market (Ball 2007). In practice, the contemporary thrust of citizenship in the context of the neo-liberal state is to increase citizens' allegiance to the state while, at the same time, fostering practices which minimize demand for state services (Hall and Coffey 2007). The thrust for the healthy citizen sits within a broader conception of citizenship comprising three dimensions: 'membership of a democratic political community; the collective benefits and rights associated with membership; and participation within the community's political, economic and social processes' (Bellamy 2008: 12).

Thus, the neo-liberal government is concerned with the varied kinds of work the rational actor does on themselves: 'social actors are induced to perform in order to comply "voluntarily" with the ends toward which their governance is directed' (Bennett *et al.* 2007: 536). According to Kelly (2006: 18):

> (Neo)Liberalism emerges, not only as a means of governing the state, the economy, and civil society, but also as a means of governing in these domains via the *rational, autonomous, responsible* behaviours and dispositions of a *free,*

prudent, active Subject: a Subject we can identify as the entrepreneurial Self. [italics in the original]

This rational, active self comes into play in advanced liberal societies as a subject who is expected to conduct himself or herself based on an ethic of active citizenship in relation to health:

> in which the maximization of lifestyle, potential, health, and quality of life has become almost obligatory, and where negative judgments are directed toward those who will not, for whatever reason, adopt an active, informed, positive, and prudent relation to the future.

(Rose 2006: 25)

In this chapter, we explore how the rational, active citizen is enmeshed in bodily practices and, more broadly, what Hohle (2009: 283) considered as 'idealized citizenship'. While Hohle was writing of Black civil rights as an embodied social movement that moulded and shaped participant bodies for political purposes, we suggest that the same may be argued in relation to physical activity and health agendas. Hohle outlined how 'citizenship schools' for Black activists sought to deracialize and thereby empower Blacks to be less Black and in turn more successful. More specifically, in Hohle's examination of citizenship schools:

> The idea was to organize a set of ethics that instructed blacks how to inspect the health of bodies – self, family, and friends – to ensure that black bodies did not conform to the black stereotypes of the dirty and unkempt self.

(Hohle 2009: 299)

As a social movement to construct and project idealized citizenship, bodily gestures, postures, grammar, habits and physical appearances were explicitly taught to urban Black people with a view to them trading their comportment for the rights and responsibilities of citizenship.

McClintock's (2009) historical research on citizenship looks at the intersection of citizenship discourses with class and, more specifically, the invention of idleness as a dimension of corporeal control. British discourses, beginning in the sixteenth century, associated poverty with the sloth of the farming classes. They functioned to 'not only to draw distinctions between labouring classes but also to sanction and enforce social discipline, to legitimize and plunder and to alter habits of labour' (p. 365), thereby socially and economically empowering those leading a particular valued 'lifestyle'. The discourses of idleness and work remain central to how the responsible (young) citizen self-manages, particularly given the co-opting of discourses of work (schoolwork, employment) to health work (diet, exercise, balance, etc.).

While studies of citizenship can highlight the significance of structural features such as race or class, according to Walkerdine (2003: 240), the neo-liberal subject is projected as one who has:

been completely freed from traditional ties of location, class and gender and to be completely self-produced. . . . Freed from ties of class the new worker is totally responsible for their own destiny and so techniques and technologies of regulation focus on the self-management of citizens to produce themselves as having the skills and qualities necessary to succeed in the new economy.

It follows that studies of citizenship also reveal shifts to a focus on 'choices' made by, and opportunities available to, citizens as individuals, rather than entitlements available from government, suggesting a more active and engaged citizenry as well as a more individual, less solidaristic, citizenship (Taylor-Gooby 2008).

In this chapter, we are interested in how young people interface with discourses around the rational, active citizen specifically in relation to physical activity and health. Following Foucault, Walkerdine (2003: 239) notes there have been 'shifts in modes of regulation [from] practices of policing and external regulation to *technologies of self-regulation* in which subjects come to understand themselves as responsible for their own regulation'. Halse (2009: 50) has built upon citizenship discourses and their contemporary features such as active citizenship and personal responsibility and proposes a notion of a 'bio-citizen' to suggest 'a new species of human being' constituted by 'welding the body onto the social, cultural, economic and political responsibilities of citizenship and the state'. She argues that '[w]hile active citizenship is central to the identity of the new bio-citizen, her/his identity also derives from the disembodied, rational subject of liberal humanism, a universal ethic of justice and a notion of the common good'. For the bio-citizen then what

> *counts* as virtuous, moral actions are those that serve the interests of the individual and all others in any society. Thus for the bio-citizen, failure to control one's weight makes one a bad citizen by ignoring the interests of the common good needed for a well-ordered society.
>
> (Halse 2009: 51)

Enacting the modes of regulation required of the new bio-citizen can be particularly intense for young people who are located within institutions of schooling and families as well as broader society. School health and physical education as well as (increasingly) health promotion in schooling and beyond seek to (re)educate young people on how to manage all aspects of their embodiment such as wearing neat school uniforms, resisting drug and alcohol abuse, managing their bodies for healthy weight and partaking in desirable socialization through sport. 'Eat well, be active' health promotion iterations are intended to be pervasive and we examine how these discourses have been taken up or resisted by the young people with whom we worked in the *Life Activity Project*.

While the health promotion literature abounds with research on how to produce compliant, risk-averse young people, relatively little is known about resistance or its potential to be generative. The young people in the *Life Activity Project* data set (aged between 12 and 20) upon which this chapter draws were similar in age to those involved in Flanagan *et al.*'s (2008) research into changes in adolescents' perceptions of their rights concerning their health and 'lifestyle' choices. They found that young people aged 14 to 15 years were more likely to argue their right to take risks with their bodies that might compromise their health and that the government had less right to constrain their individual choices i.e. personal rights peaked around 14–15 years old. That said, females were less likely to endorse individual rights and more likely to endorse public health messages. Thus, we are interested in patterns of resistance, perhaps seen as an individual's 'right', as well as compliance and structural features that may moderate accessing 'healthy lifestyles'.

The slim, mesomorphic, physically active, fruit and vegetable consuming body is said to symbolize a particular idealized citizen constructed discursively, corporeally and performatively (Hohle 2009). As will be seen in the data to follow, young peoples' techniques of self management (i.e. resources employed to work on the body to meet citizenship expectations) were differently known, valued, available, managed, taken up and associated with both pleasure and pain. Hall and Coffey (2007: 294) reminds us that citizenship 'figures as a language of both anxiety and aspiration'. Walkerdine (2003: 241) explains:

> The issue is that, in the Foucauldian sense, the practices of subjectification produce a constantly failing subject who has to understand their position in essentially personal and psychological terms. It is, of course a deep irony that the subject of neo-liberalism is actually produced as multiple, having to cope with existing in a number of different discourses and positions: the subject who is supposed to be able to choose who they are from a myriad of offerings, who can make themselves.

Our analysis of citizenship anxieties and aspirations draws on the *Life Activity Project* data set. As outlined in Chapter 1, it comprises a series of interviews, across a number of years, with purposively selected young people from across the eastern states of Australia. An analysis of data entered into QSR Nvivo under nodes such as 'knowing the right thing', 'health, 'fun', 'care', 'I should' and 'time management' was conducted to identify common themes and language use.

The first section of the chapter then looks at what information (and misinformation) the young people 'know' constitutes an appropriate 'lifestyle' and how these messages should be played out in their own lives. The corollary is the value that the young people place on particular corporeal practices within their daily lives. The second section focuses on the feelings of guilt and disappointment associated with living up (or not) to what the young people know and value, while the third section looks at the pervasiveness of the individual's sense of responsibility to live the discourses, despite structural and contextual barriers and tensions.

Knowing and valuing healthy citizenship

The aforementioned theoretical frameworks suggest the starting point for active citizenship is to know and understand the 'rules', to understand what it is one should do to be a 'good citizen'. The second requirement is to understand that following the rules is imperative to being a good citizen and contributing to the good of society. While the first was very evident in the data, the second was more subtly embedded in *how* the young people talked about health and how people *should* behave; it was more about what was taken-for-granted as normative behaviour rather than explicitly expressed as contributing or not to the common good.

We can say with some conviction that the most of the young people in the study no matter what their class or gender, *knew* what it meant to be a healthy person in ways espoused in public health policy, health promotion strategies and school curricula (Baum 2008). As is evident from other chapters in this section of the book, an understanding of health as eating the right kinds of foods (primarily vegetables and fruit), avoiding 'fast foods' and food high in sugar and fat and engaging in sufficient physical activity to maintain the balance of energy in energy out, was something they all offered as central to being healthy. For some this was complemented by references to emotional, social and mental health. But even when these other elements were mentioned, balancing intake of food and expenditure of energy still dominated most descriptions of health and featured as the primary areas which required attention if the participants saw themselves as needing to be more healthy.

The following quotes are typical of responses to questions about the participants' meanings of health or about how they would rate their health (from 1, poor, to 10, the best). For example, in the following quote, although Faye begins by associating health with a psychological attribute, she soon moves on to defining health in terms of food and exercise:

> Well I think that confidence is a good think, but also to be aware of um, you know, eating the right thing, but also not trying to diet. Like not trying to cut back on what you eat but eating healthier and also do lots of exercise.
>
> (Faye, interview 2000)

In one of his early interviews, Felippe rated his health '3, 4, 4 to the max'. When asked what he would need to do to be healthier, he replied: 'Not be physically inactive, eat healthy, eat like no fatty foods, I eat like ten eggs a week and just my eating habits are not very good, high in fat' (Felippe, interview 2001).

It was also well understood that if one practised unhealthy behaviours (if one were 'inactive' or ate the wrong foods) one would suffer the consequences now and in the future. For some of the participants, the consequences were clearly in relation to appearance, for others the threat of ill-health and even not getting a job. This quote from Felicia, also illustrates how parents' comments were often important in presenting the consequences of 'unhealthy' behaviour:

> My parents are always saying 'eat healthy because you don't want to, by the age of twenty-six, you don't want to be really, really big and not be able to do anything'. You see a lot of places when you go for jobs and they don't accept like bigger people. It's been on the news a couple of times and they were having like anti-discrimination or something like that, which there's a policy on.

> . . . I think it helps you, I think perhaps you'll live longer, the healthier you are, the better life you'll have to live; longer lasting. I think it's important.
>
> (Felicia, interview 2001)

This notion of responsibility, an understanding of what it takes to be a 'good' citizen and how to assess oneself as such, manifested in the young peoples' talk as imperatives, this is what one (any 'responsible person') *should* do. For example, in the following quote Eun-ji, in defining 'being healthy' in terms of eating health foods and exercising, that is, 'balancing energy in and out' (the key tenets of a 'healthy lifestyle'), reiterates that this is something you/one *should* do, *have to* do; to not do so is unthinkable. She directly addresses the irresponsible person who might transgress this rule: 'If you do eat fatty foods don't just sit around and do nothing'. If you can't manage this you should at least try – to not 'try' from this discursive position is to have given up on being a 'good' person.

> Being fit and not eating fatty foods or if you do eat fatty foods you *have to* burn them off. If you do eat fatty foods *don't* just sit around and do nothing. You *have to* exercise and keep it off and have like, because we go shopping every Friday and I usually get chips every Friday it's just like a treat once a week. . . . [And you reckon you have to burn those off over the weekend] Yep. And if you can't do that *try not* to have so much fatty foods and stuff.
>
> (Eun-ji, interview 2002, italics to indicate imperatives)

Although the descriptions of lives over time demonstrated quite clearly how the capacity to manage their own health was substantially constrained by financial and geographical factors and competing family, health, study and work priorities, most of the young people still blamed themselves for failing to eat and exercise in the ways they 'knew' they should (see Chapter 10). Even those who resisted the imperative, for example, to 'be active', knew that they *should* be more active and judged themselves accordingly, some being more sanguine about this than others.

Angela, for example, is quite clear in the following quote that being physically active is not at all on her mind. Angela's comment is reminiscent of the responses of the African American young women to similar questions, in their case about food (in Chapter 11). Her own background is Fijian Indian and this culture seems to play a role in her capacity to challenge the discourse – few other participants in the studies would have been able or wanted to represent themselves in this way. On the other hand, she recognizes herself as a 'bad' citizen, but she is not too worried about it and suggests that it is no one else's business. The following quote begins with her response to a question about 'how she sees fitness?'

Angela: Okay, firstly the word fitness, anyway, the first image I would get in my head would be like people exercising, running around, doing weights or whatever. So again I'd be like 'nah, wrong direction, don't want to see that word, moving on'.

Int: How do you think about yourself as in taking care of yourself?

Angela:	Out of ten I would probably give it three.
Int:	Why is that, what do you mean by that?
Angela:	Well, I'm aware that I don't take care of myself that well. I'm a junk food junkie big time; chips [. . .] like in that aspect I know that what I'm doing is not right, it's not healthy and I'm not getting fit or anything. But even knowing that, it's not stopping me, I'm like, okay, I know that but I don't care, why should anyone else, I won't stop doing it, so, in that way I suppose, I'm not really all that, looking after myself that well, in the health and fitness way.

(Angela, interview 2002)

For Angela her priorities lie elsewhere with completing college so that she can earn money and be independent and with her relationships with friends and family. She simply does not subscribe to a discourse which suggests she is not a good citizen if she does not eat well and exercise.

> So I don't really have a priority at the moment. But I guess getting through college is one of my priorities. . . . I guess, college would be my first and my friends would be, well, my social life would be my second, yeah and then somewhere down there is my family.

(Angela, interview 2002)

For most of the young men in the *Life Activity Project*, if they were involved in physical activity and most were, it was mostly about the enjoyment afforded by playing sport with others, being skilled or being fit enough to play sport or to feel capable. It wasn't until sport was no longer organized for them at school, or they began to feel they wanted to look better, be more physical/masculine, that they began to be more reflective about their 'lifestyles'. Steve's example, however, suggests that for some at least, messages about health were not completely absent in their thinking about how they should conduct their lives. In the following quote, Steve begins by suggesting that he is pretty laid-back, a bit of a lounge lizard, but then goes on to say that he regularly walks six kilometres and that he does this for 'health and fitness'; one year later, Steve has a personal trainer who instructs him on good eating as well as physical fitness. This was explained in terms of improving his body shape so that he was more muscular ('less skinny'). In none of Steve's talk, and this is typical of most of the young men's talk, is there any mention of 'guilt' or 'laziness' or 'anxiety'.

Steve:	Weekends, just the activities, I normally go to the beach and will just lounge around the house watching movies and stuff or Friday nights, sometimes I'll go and watch my sister play sport. I'll sit and watch her and [. . .]
Int:	You don't do sport at all.
Steve:	No, no, very little exercise.
Int:	Why is that?
Steve:	I've never been a really sporty person. I'll go out for a walk of a night time which is a fair distance and then walk back.

Int: How far would you walk of a night time?
Steve: About six k's.
Int: Why do you do that?
Steve: Just to make sure I'm fit and healthy.

(Steve, interview 2004)

Not measuring up: guilt and anxiety

In contrast to Steve's comments, for many of the young women, particularly the middle-class urban young women, health was about balancing energy in and energy out so that they were comfortable with the way they looked (see also Chapters 5 and 10; Wright *et al.* 2006). In the context of the bio-citizen, to look fat or overweight is to demonstrate your incapacity to care for yourself; to be a good citizen is to eat well and exercise or at least to burn off what you have eaten if you have transgressed. Being healthy or rather not being healthy as indicated by over-weight or even potential overweight was thus closely associated with feelings of guilt and anxiety. For many of the young people, and mostly the young women, this was much more likely appear in conversations where they talked about their own experiences (rather than how others *should* behave), often in terms of their failure to manage their eating and exercise in ways that they feel they should. Such talk was usually accompanied by self-designations of being lazy and feelings of guilt. These feelings were experienced viscerally, they were embodied in ways variously described as feeling 'bad', 'sluggish', 'oily' or 'missing something'. For example, in explaining how she feels if she misses a gym class, Jessica says: 'I will feel bad. I would feel guilty. Yeah, I feel like I'm obligated. It's personal. Like to keep going and get fit. Stop being so lazy.' Concomitantly, being active and managing the bal-ance between energy in and energy out produced good feelings, feelings that for some were also associated with being productive and 'not wasting time':

> Because then I feel better about myself [if I exercise] and in the end I feel better overall in terms of like my body, like it feels better, it feels stronger . . . Because [if you sit in front of the TV] you just feel like you've done nothing, like you've wasted you time.

(Faye, interview 2000)

For Chrissie, not being active is much more about her anxieties about her appear-ance, about putting on weight and the bad feelings that come from that. These bad feelings, however, are not simply about what she looks like but are embodied, if she is not active, she feels 'like something is missing'. The imperative has been inter-nalized, if she does not eat well and active, she will suffer (feel bad and possibly put on weight). In the following quote, she has just been asked how she knows if she is healthy and if she pays any attention to health messages. Her first response is to say that she knows by just looking at herself and then she thinks what I *have to* do. This is then followed by talk about the pleasure and positive feelings of having more energy she derives from body combat, followed again by the bad feelings she has if she eats badly and does not exercise. The feeling bad does not seem to match the missing out of the fun of body combat – it is not simply missing the pleasure of the activity or even not feeling so energetic – but one of suffering and guilt.

> No, not really, I just look at myself and think what I have to do, like with body combat it's so much fun and I feel like I have more energy and think I should keep doing it because if I stop I'm just gonna lose all that and I don't want to lose all that and it's like a form of exercise and it's fun. But I just think if I eat badly, if I don't do exercise, I don't do this, I'm the one who is gonna suffer and no one else.
>
> (Chrissie, interview 2003)

Again in another response in the same interview, the same mixture of talk about the embodied pleasure from exercise and guilt and moral self-judgement (being a couch potato) is evident when Chrissie is asked, why she would continue going to the gym:

Chrissie: um to keep the whole exercise, fit, routine going. So you're not, like because I'm not going to the gym I feel sort of, um, not sluggish, but *like some thing is missing*. Like at the moment it's all schoolwork and you sort of need a break so I've just started taking my dog for a walk around the block. It's just some exercise. It's just something that gets me out of the house and gets me moving because *I don't want to turn into a couch potato* right before the formal and I don't want to have to get another dress because I have put on too much weight, . . .

Int: How do you think your health is in all of this?

Chrissie: I think it is a lot better now; not a lot better but because I'm going to the gym every week, I haven't missed a week. We normally go Mondays and Wednesdays and if I miss one day I'll make it up during the week so I still go the same amount, because if I don't, I feel very guilty. I feel guilty and I feel really good after I go to the gym because it's a relief and you do the exercise and I really enjoy it, it's fun and it's hanging out with your friends too and it's good.

(Chrissie, interview 2003)

Appearance was monitored by looking in the mirror and through the fit of clothes, but some of the young women also regularly monitored their weight by standing on the scales. For Natasha this is a daily regime, one clearly fraught with anxiety and frustration:

Natasha: I look in the mirror and I think oh my god and I'm really paranoid about it because I don't want to, I've been trying really hard to lose it and I can't, like I stopped eating all the shit and I'm doing all the exercise, like I did a two hour walk today and in the last couple of days I've been doing walking . . .

Int: Do you actually weigh yourself?
Natasha: Every day.
Int: So you have scales and you weigh yourself every day.
Natasha: Yeah just like I'll drink water and I have a salad and I put on three kilos.

(Natasha, interview 2004)

The ideal citizen: doing it alone?

Across the *Life Activity Project* cohorts, family priorities, configurations and resources in the form of time, money, transport, etc. were expended by the 'good parent/citizen' to provide activity-rich contexts for their children (see also Macdonald *et al.* 2004). A parent interviewed in Lee's (2005) study captures the extent of this commitment:

Int: So how are you involved in the children's activities?
Mother: I drive them everywhere, I make them lunches if they're swimming and they've got to go to somewhere after I usually make them a pasta dish and keep their energy levels high. Especially with Brandon, I mean there was one stage where we were picking him up from swimming, he had half an hour to have something to eat and we'd drop him off at [touch] football and he wouldn't get home until Monday night about eight o'clock. And yeah, same with when they finish school of an afternoon they usually walk up to the pool and I usually make sure that they've got extras packed in their lunch box kind of thing food-wise. What else do I do with them?
Int: You said that you both go down to the swimming club and help out with the club and that sort of thing?
Mother: Yeah and with Friday night is a thing where we go to swimming club . . . and Terrence [husband] helps with the barbeque or whatever you know.
Int: And actually I talked with Brandon about the volleyball and you do a bit of car pooling and that sort of thing?
Mother: . . . On Wednesday afternoons if they go to another school because we've got a Tarago [van] kind of thing we can just about get the whole team in, so we can take the whole team in one go.
Int: Okay so that's your biggest role, with transport?
Mother: Yeah, transport, transport would be our biggest role yes.

(Brandon's mother, parent interview 2003)

Thus, for some young people, their families were invested in physical activity and diet regimes (see Felicia before) consistent with the bio-citizen.

Kendra, on the other hand, attended a school in a rural town and for the interview period was either living by herself or with her boyfriend because of abusive relationships in her own family. The way Kendra, however, talks about her life draws very much on discourses of self-responsibility – she is literally independent, she has to make her own way and part of that, from her point of view, is taking responsibility for her own health and weight. Unlike Chrissie, Faye and Eun-ji and many of the other young people in the study, Kendra's only option was walking, school-based physical activity and housework, she could not afford to go to the gym and did not have the resources or support for community sport or physical activity. On one hand, she was the ideal neo-liberal subject, on the other she was very vulnerable taking full responsibility for making her own life. In the following section, she is describing how she used to be fat and therefore stopped doing PE at her old school, but has begun again at her new school.

Int: Could you explain that kind of view of yourself? Like you went from being very physical activity, very physically active into inactivity.

Kendra: I didn't like it. I feel better about myself now being physical and being able to do stuff with myself. Eating healthy, trying to get myself back on track. To what I used to be. Like I hated it. I didn't like being the way I was. Because I wasn't active, I didn't do nothing. I just sat around, ate food all the time. Didn't do nothing. Now I feel, I go to school, I get up every morning and feel really good about myself and stuff. It's good.

Int: Can you pinpoint or recognise a point in time when things changed for you? Was there anybody that encouraged you or changed things?

Kendra: No, well I got kicked out of home. I quit school and then come back. Because I used to go school over in S. . . . But I just didn't do it and over here it's different again. But yeah I just got back into gear and thought this is ridiculous. I don't like being fat and nobody likes me and everyone used to pick on me. So I thought I'll just get back into it. And I used to walk everywhere, never sat down. I just walked . . . all the time. I just go back into it.

(Kendra, interview 2001)

However, for Kendra, like many of the other rural young people and the young Muslim women in Knez's study (see Chapter 8), school provides the only form of accessible purposive recreational physical activity. Dance, which she loves doing at school was only available in another town and not accessible without a car or family to drive her there.

Now we [she and her boyfriend] have broken up and stuff and when I am home by myself I don't just sit there. I clean up the house, vacuum the floors or put some music on and I like to dance so I stay in my bedroom and dance and work up a sweat so I think that is about my physical activity. . . .

(Kendra, interview 2002)

Underpinning Kendra's responses was the assumption that individuals were responsible for managing their own health. Rachel (interview 2002) says explicitly: 'Yeah, I mean we're ultimately in control of ourselves I reckon. I mean if we want to we can and if we want to do exercise we can; yeah, it's all about, I don't know [laughs].'

Kendra was not alone in her vulnerability. Jessica Lee's (2004) study of rural young people illustrates how tensions between the ideal citizen and barriers to meeting this ideal became more pronounced as family circumstances changed. For example, Wadiken's daily routines changed as the drought hit the family farm and he and his siblings were required to work on handfeeding the cattle and sheep. At a more mundane level, many participants cited the lack of access to transport as prohibiting their participation in many of the activities they enjoyed, particularly organized sport. Despite these life-changing circumstances, the young people often continued to explain their capacity to engage in physical activity in terms of their own strengths or failings. They held themselves responsible for not being as active as they thought they should be.

Conclusion

'Good citizens are clean, healthy, strong, and fit rather than dirty, sick, weak, and fat' (Hohle 2009: 300). It follows that this good (bio-) citizen is then in a position to contribute towards the common good (Halse 2009). Young people in the *Life Activity Project* and its adjunct projects had learnt this. More specifically, they knew the prescription: exercise enough not to get fat, eat food that will not make you fat or exercise to balance food intake. Like research conducted in the broader field of citizenship (e.g. Flanagan *et al.* 2008; Sherrod 2008), the young people in the *Life Activity Project* frequently approached living out this script as a civic responsibility they held and infrequently questioned the explicit and subtle technologies employed by the neo-liberal state to promote particular individual choices in the interests of public health. Data supported the argument that cultural shifts in citizenship and their interplay with health and education have influenced how young people think about their behaviour and the 'right way' to act or contemplate acting. In this chapter, we have argued that for many young people physical activity and health practices constitute a symbolic citizenship, embodied as healthy weight, slim/muscular body shape, physically active, ready-for-work and disciplined. Thus, a good citizen is one who knows the facts, self-assesses, self-monitors and acts (or knows to express self-disappointments should they fail to act).

The normative frameworks in shaping and giving meaning to young people's perspectives and choices were bound up with their social interactions with, for example, the school curriculum, peers, family and media that nourished and sustained adherence. For some, the family worked to ensure regimes around physical activity and food consumption were consistent with 'good parenting' and, in turn, healthy citizenship. There were also many young people who worked somewhat alone at mastering 'healthy' techniques of self and this became more apparent as participants aged. What was shared, however, was the constant physical, social and emotional work entailed in being or becoming a healthy citizen. Even resistance to the dominant discourse was deliberative and, for some, emotionally draining given the associated guilt.

With the strong sense of individual responsibility for healthy citizenship rather than state, the *Life Activity Project*'s participants had little sense of their citizen entitlements or rights in relation to access and equity. One exception was Felicia, a mother of four young children living in marginal, working-class area. Here she refuses to take responsibility for social and structural aspects of her environment which differentiate her chances of engaging herself and her children in physical activity and 'good' eating.

> Well they come in saying they are going to snatch people's children away because they are obese. But you don't see them trying to help families out. They could help families and stuff; they could give some benefits to [to families] for transport. Single mothers get cheaper transport; they get concessions. They don't pay anything to the RTA [Roads and Traffic Authority] for registering their car. . . . But with health you don't see anything with health; you don't get a discount at the gym; you don't get a discount at the swimming pool. If you want to put your son in swim classes or your daughter in swim classes you don't get that discount. It's like why is it different for everything else when everyone uses it. I guess like with groceries and stuff it would help out. The people who have money, have nice stuff, have nice clothes, have educated kids, upper class schools, they don't struggle whatsoever. And then you see families that have lower incomes, struggling, working, twice as much overtime and they still have barely enough to survive to put their kids into things like swimming classes, gymnastics and dance and art school. It's just not fair. People living in [urban fringe] compared to people living in the city get treated very differently, very differently. I think it's rude to be honest.
>
> (Felicia, interview 2007)

The rarity of this response underscores the ways most of the young people in the study took on self-responsibility for being active, consistent with neo-liberal discourses of the sovereignty of aspiration, personal choice and consumption (Taylor-Gooby 2008; Walkerdine 2003).

The social and political forces associated with bio-citizenship remind us that citizenship education is not limited to school-based subject matter circumscribed as history or civics but is enmeshed across the curriculum, co-curricular activities, the media, etc. as young people are exposed to a citizenship education that values a healthy, informed and physically active citizen (Pike 2007), and, more generally, how citizenship is powerfully embodied. Interestingly, while ethnic and cultural differences and their articulation with citizenship challenges governments the world over (Bellamy 2008), the symbolic citizenship of having or aspiring to a healthy (thin), active body was common across the diverse groups of young people with whom we worked (see chapters in this section for the similarity of discourses employed by young people from a range of socio-economic status, geographical locations and ethnicities).

We note, however, that the healthy citizen was predominantly delimited to diet and exercise. While this may have been, in part, a result of the sequence of questions and interviews, there was scope for participants to take a broader view of health. It raises interesting questions as to how the hegemony of these particular discourses has come to be across such a breadth of contexts. Perhaps even more interesting is how, given the cognizance and verbal commitment of young people to these discourses, governments worldwide are concerned and baffled that the diet/exercise prescription is 'not working'. We are also left with questions that take us back to the notion of a (politically) active citizen and what an empowered citizenry might look like with respect to young people's physical activity and health. What would be the physical activity and health priorities and behaviours of a truly active, informed citizenry? How would such a citizenry come to be? What would be the impact on public policy and provision or, indeed, the media? We leave you, the reader, with these questions to take up in your own research.

References

Ball, S. J. (2007) *Education PLC: understanding private sector participation in public sector education*, London: Routledge.

Baum, F. (2008) *The New Public Health*, Melbourne: Oxford University Press.

Bellamy, R. (2008) *Citizenship: a very short introduction*, New York: Oxford University Press.

Bennett, T., Dodsworth, F. and Joyce, P. (2007) 'Introduction – liberalism, government, culture', *Cultural Studies*, 21(4–5): 525–48.

Flanagan, C. A., Stout, M. and Gallay, L. S. (2008) 'It's my body and none of your business: developmental changes in adolescents' perceptions of rights concerning health', *Journal of Social Issues*, 64(4): 815–34.

Hall, T. and Coffey, A. (2007) 'Learning selves and citizenship: gender and youth transitions', *Journal of Social Policy*, 36(2): 279–96.

Halse, C. (2009) 'Bio-citizenship: virtue discourses and the birth of the bio-citizen', in J. Wright and V. Harwood (eds) *Biopolitics and the 'Obesity Epidemic': governing bodies*, New York: Routledge.

Hohle, R. (2009) 'The body and citizenship in social movement research: embodied performances and the deracialized self in the Black Civil Rights Movement 1961–65', *The Sociological Quarterly*, 50(2): 283–307.

Kelly, P. (2006) 'The entrepreneurial self and "youth at-risk": exploring the horizons of identity in the twenty-first century', *Journal of Youth Studies*, 9(1): 17–32.

Lee, J. (2005) *Physical Activity and Physical Culture in the Lives of Rural Young People*, Brisbane: The University of Queensland.

McClintock, A. (2009) 'The white family of man', in L. Black and J. Solomos (eds) *Theories of Race and Racism*, London: Routledge.

Macdonald, D., Rodger, S., Ziviani, J., Jenkins, D., Batch, J. and Jones, J. (2004) 'Physical activity as a dimension of family life for lower primary school children', *Sport, Education and Society*, 9(3): 307–26.

Pike, M. A. (2007) 'The state and citizenship education in England: a curriculum for subjects or citizens?', *Journal of Curriculum Studies*, 39(4): 471–89.

Rose, N. (2006) *The Politics of Life Itself: biopower and subjectivity in the twenty-first century*, Princeton, NJ: Princeton University Press.

Sherrod, L. R. (2008) 'Adolescents' perceptions of rights as reflected in their views of citizenship', *Journal of Social Issues*, 64(4): 771–90.

Sinclair, J. (1818) *The Code of Health and Longevity*, London: Macmillan.

Taylor-Gooby, P. (2008) *Reframing Social Citizenship*, New York: Oxford University Press.

Walkerdine, V. (2003) 'Reclassifying upward mobility: femininity and the neo-liberal subject', *Gender and Education*, 15(3): 237–48.

Wright, J., O'Flynn, G. and Macdonald, D. (2006) 'Being fit and looking healthy: young women's and men's constructions of health and fitness', *Sex Roles*, 54(9–10): 707–16.

10 Young people, transitions and physical activity

Jan Wright and Judy Laverty

In the literature on young people's health and its relation to participation in physical activity, there are recurring narratives that lament the decline in participation during the senior years of schooling and beyond (e.g. Sallis *et al.* 2000). This apparent decline has been interpreted as a significant problem and one that must be addressed by strategies to engage young people in more physical activity; most of which target young people with a view to changing their attitudes and behaviours (Gyurcsik *et al.* 2004; Leslie *et al.* 2001). This concern about young people's participation in physical activity seems to be embedded in, and adds support to, a notion that adolescence is a developmental period of 'increased risk', where young people are particularly susceptible to, and held responsible for, making 'bad' health choices (Rose 1992), as parents and schools exert a diminished influence over their lives.

In this chapter, we do not debate that having the opportunity to be active, in a range of different ways and for a range of reasons, is not the 'right' of every young person. For many of the young people in our study being able to engage in physical activity brought a great deal of pleasure, satisfaction and feelings of well-being to their lives. What we will argue in this chapter, however, is that 'choices' about physical activity (like other choices being made in the years immediately after school) are made in a complex environment, where young people are attempting to negotiate new expectations and work and/or study often takes priority (White and Wyn 2004). What we *do* want to do is offer a response to current research and policy which does not seem to take this into account; we want to offer an understanding of physical activity participation as complex and situated, as embedded in social processes and structures, which have sustained effects on the decisions young people make and how they think about themselves and their lives. We want to contribute to policy and planning in ways that take into account these complexities, that improve lives and 'resist . . . [the] reductive urge towards universality and essentialism' (Slee 2000: xi), which currently characterizes the policy around physical activity and health.

To do this we take a sociological approach to youth which points to the importance of understanding young people's lives and how these are 'constructed and shaped by institutional processes and social structures and by individuals and groups' (White and Wyn 2004: vii). A feature of recent writing on young people drawing on such an approach is the notion that in contemporary societies, where life trajectories are increasingly unpredictable and uncertain, much of the responsibility 'for negotiating their own life patterns' (Winter and Stone 1999, quoted in Abbott-Chapman 2000: 21) is left to young people (Fitzclarence 2004; White and Wyn 2004). From this point of view, 'choices' around leisure and health are important in how young people constitute their own biographies (Beck and Beck-Gernsheim 2002). As we will demonstrate later 'choices', however, are not equally distributed and, for some of the young people in the *Life Activity Project*, their 'choices' were considerably constrained by economic and social circumstances.

This chapter then will use the narratives of the young people in the *Life Activity Project* to explore the changing place and meanings of physical activity for young people as they make 'choices' about their lives during and beyond school. The young people who feature in this chapter are those for whom we have data from interviews in their last years of schooling – that is, from Years 10/11 (when they were 15–17 years of age) to their final year – and then again from recent interviews when they were 20–24 years of age. For some of the NSW cohort, there are also interviews in the intervening years. Unfortunately we were unable to re-establish contact with the Victorian cohort for the longitudinal study once they left school, which is why they have not been included in this chapter. The variability in numbers of male and female participants is a consequence we would argue of this kind of qualitative study: the young women were more amenable to ongoing contact and in NSW were also part of a doctoral study which meant they had established stronger links with the project.

The young people featured in this chapter come from five of the schools in the project: Malcos, the elite independent boys' school (five young men) and Bloomsbury, the elite independent girls' school (six young women); Seachrist College, the non-elite Catholic high school situated in a regional coastal city (one young man and three young women); and the two government schools – Sunnydale, on the urban fringes of a large city (two young men and five young women) and Greenvalley, the semi-rural school (one young man and two young women). Although in this chapter we are using the elite independent schools as markers of social class, we want to be clear that some of the young people who attend these schools, and indeed several of the young people we interviewed, came from backgrounds that were far from affluent. For these young people, both parents worked long hours specifically to support their children at the schools. However, what has been interesting to us is how the values/dispositions (habitus) inculcated by the school took hold across the group, no matter what their parents' socio-economic status.

Theorizing young people, transitions and choice biographies

The term 'transition' has been commonly used as an economic concept to describe the move by young people from school into the labour force. Transition studies have traditionally used age as a critical marker of change and infer that young people make a linear, permanent progression through different life and/or career stages. Wyn and Woodman (2006) argue the transitions experienced by baby boomers (including school to work shifts, leaving home and establishing nuclear families) have become the dominant way of describing how younger generations make a life, even though these transitions reflect particular historical and cultural influences. This conceptualization has been criticized by youth researchers because it assumes that youth is simply a 'transitional stage' between childhood and the independence of adult life. White and Wyn (2004: 8) argue that 'this approach conflates youth development processes with social processes; it generally assumes a linear trajectory and makes normative assumptions about young people's lives'.

Using data from the *Life Patterns Research Project*, White and Wyn (2004) draw attention to the more complex processes of transitions evident in the lives of young people in both rural and urban areas of Victoria, who were often simultaneously working and studying. Related studies by Wyn and Woodman (2006) also illustrate how young people's pathways are more complicated. They found young people constructed pathways that reflected a complex mix of leaving and returning home, undertaking part-time and full-time work at different stages and in some cases, undertaking full-time study and full-time work.

From these and other studies (e.g. Ball *et al.* 2000), it is possible to see how linear constructions of transition appear to be increasingly out of step and almost irrelevant to some young people's lives. As Wyn and Dwyer point out, these studies indicate:

> that many in the younger generation are becoming increasingly pro-active in the face of risk and uncertainty of outcomes, and are making pragmatic choices for themselves which enable them to maintain their aspirations despite the persistence of structural influences on their lives.
>
> (Wyn and Dwyer 1999: 5)

At the same time, social theorists have also suggested that young people today, living in societies influenced by the 'political and economic culture of neo-liberalism', have had to come to understand themselves as able to make their own futures and as responsible for the choices they make in this process. This process has been described as one of 'individualization', where individuals are increasingly held 'accountable for their own survival in a time where change is the only certainty' (Ball *et al.* 2000: 2). And as Ball *et al.* (2000) found, young people do see themselves as being in charge of their own destinies no matter what their life circumstances:

> In all of the recent major studies of youth transitions from school to work, as with our own one consistent finding emerges . . . Young people constantly reiterate that they do have choices, that luck, hard work and sheer determination are the bases of 'success' . . . The young people in our study were most likely to blame themselves for any lack of success, either because of stress or failure to 'see their best interests'.
>
> (Ball *et al.* 2000: 4)

While Ball is talking primarily about success in relation to work and post-school study, the same might be said of young people's participation in physical activity.

In relation to the discourse that suggests good citizens have a moral obligation to be physically active for their health, the young people often blamed themselves for their perceived inactivity, despite their narratives demonstrating that the circumstances of their lives made finding time and energy for physical activity beyond the demands of work extremely difficult.

As those writing about young people's choices from a socially critical perspective demonstrate, 'choices' are made in relation to experiences (biographies) and the social, cultural and economic context in which the young people live. As Ball *et al.* (2000: 150), talking more specifically about the role of space and time, conclude from their study 'the geographies and other possibilities for identity are not the same for all', nor are they stable and unchanging. Some identities are more fragile and some more stable or secure. This is discussed further in their detailed interpretation of young people's narratives in their book, *Choice, Pathways and Transitions Post-16* (Ball *et al.* 2000). However, what we have taken from their analysis is the notion of identities as a shifting framework for making choices. For Ball and his colleagues, the interest was in 'learning identities' and their connection with young people's choices in relation to post-school education. We propose the notion of 'physical activity identities' to help understand the interaction between young people's histories and their social, cultural, economic and, in our case, geographical environments, as they make choices about physical activity beyond school.

The term 'learning identities' as used by Ball *et al.* (2000) has come from an exploration of a sociology of lifelong learning by Rees *et al.* (1997). 'Learning identities', according to Rees *et al.* (1997: 493), is a concept that captures a number of ideas: 'learning identities' serve as the framework individuals use to view learning and for making decisions about it; they are 'essentially personal with emotional as well as intellectual dimensions'; but they are also products of social experience (that is, of interactions with institutions, places, discourses/ideas, etc.).

For our purposes then, 'physical activity identities' are identities which are shaped through individuals' interactions with informal and formal lived experiences of physical activity; interactions which are likely to be associated with particular emotions – pleasurable and unpleasurable – and to have left indelible traces that continue to influence their identities. Physical activity identities are also formed through interactions with particular knowledge or ideas about physical activity (for example, discourses about its relationship to health, to lifestyles and to productive citizenship). Physical activity identities become 'frameworks' for how potential physical activity participation is viewed/evaluated and for making decisions about it. In this chapter we explore how particular physical activity identities are shaped by the experiences of physical activity during the school years (but not necessarily at school) and how they then come into play in decisions made about physical activity post-school.

Transitions for the young people in the *Life Activity Project* (LAP)

We use the term 'transition' in the chapter to describe the complex process of moving beyond a time when school is a major organizing feature of the LAP young people's lives. On one hand, there was a very clear notion that they had come to the end of a particular time in their lives, a time when the structure of schooling dominated the way they organized their lives. For most, however, this did not signal a transition from school to paid work; paid work had been part of their lives from 14 or 15 years of age and leaving school meant either increased hours or the reorganization of work around study at vocational colleges or university. As White and Wyn (2004: 173) point out, '[f]or young people, paid work is very often a necessity – in terms of supplementing incomes, of vocational and workplace experiences, and with regard to maintaining group friendships and peer networks'. Most of their part-time work was casual, poorly paid, but necessary to maintain the levels of independence that the young people sought, even when, or perhaps because, they were living at home.

Post-school study in the three years directly after school was one of the main differentiating features of the groups: all of the young people from the elite independent schools were studying at university or had taken a 'gap' year before beginning their study; only one of the young women in the study from the government and coast schools achieved her goal of direct university entry. For those who had hoped for university (and many had), but not achieved a high enough score, most began studying at Technical and Further Education (TAFE) or a similar vocational college, some with a view of reapplying to university when they completed their diplomas. The remainder extended their work hours at their current jobs, took on extra jobs or explored different configurations of work.

The young people from the elite private schools, like the middle-class participants in Ball *et al.*'s (2000) study, talked about their lives in terms of choices made to balance leisure and pleasure with study and work. All of the young people, however, talked about their lives as 'made' by their own choices and decisions. There were, however, few certain futures and from one interview to another the young people had often made new choices because of unpredictable events (such as scores too low to get into preferred courses of study, health issues, childbirth, new opportunities for careers and new partners). At the same time they imagined themselves in futures with partners and children.

School physical activity and physical activity identities

Physical activity identities like learning identities are contingent on experiences and the relationship between these and social context and, for the young people in our study, geographical context. For the young people from the elite schools, their schools placed immense value on physical activity as contributing to the wider goals of the school, and set up expectations, structures and resources to support this (see, for example, Wright and O'Flynn 2007, and Chapter 5). The effects of such investments and expectations were strikingly evident in the ways the young people from these schools talked about physical activity and the place of it in their lives. Physical activity was inculcated as a 'disposition' essential to a 'normal, full life'. There was a subtle gender dimension to this: for the young women it was more likely to be associated with maintaining an acceptable weight (see Wright *et al.*

2006), for the young men it was part of being accepted as a male member of the student body. This is made explicit in the following quote from Aidan who represented the school in soccer, cricket and Australian Rules Football: 'I've always done them [his sports], if you know what I mean. And just a chance to go out with your mates and also, I mean if you don't play anything at school you're a nobody' (Aidan, interview 2001).

For the young people from the government and coast schools, where school-based ideas about physical activity were embedded in discourses of health, enjoyment and lifelong physical activity (see Wright and O'Flynn 2007); practices were more haphazard and more reliant on individual interest for engagement. There was neither the level of resources nor the tailoring of physical activity to their interests evident in the elite schools. For the students from the coast school, the surf, the beach and (for the female students) organized sport were reasonably accessible and generally played some part in the young people's lives, irrespective of family income. For the young men in particular, and Rusty is a good example, their physical activity identities were constituted in relation to the beach and to the physical environment. While organized sport such as rugby league, within or outside of school, was also part of their lives, they had often begun surfing at an early age. Even when this was associated with institutional settings such as surf club, being able to surf contributed to shaping a particular form of physical activity identity (or rather a 'surfer identity') that was less reliant on opportunities provided, or mediated by institutions or commercial or community providers.

For the young women on the coast, surfing was also a possibility but less likely than for the young men on the coast. While the beach (and surf clubs) provided one option, their physical activity was more likely to be mediated by school, sports clubs or community providers (commercial and otherwise). The range of these available within their locality was quite broad and accessible. For example, Tamara described herself in her early interviews as someone who had always been into physical activity: she started swimming, ballet and gymnastics very young. In her Year 10 interview she was still managing to fit in squad training and surf club, competitive acrobatics and tae kwon do, while also working at two jobs after school and on the weekend. Later interviews suggest that for Tamara at least part of her need to do some kind of physical activity was associated with her concern to maintain or reduce her weight. During her school interviews, Tamara found it difficult to imagine not being active in some way:

Int: Why do you have to do it, do you have to do it because of training or because of competition or because you just have to do it?

Tamara: Everything, I need to do something, I can't not do anything, I need to, you feel funny.

(Tamara, interview Year 10 2001)

For the young people at Sunnydale, ethnicity, as well as gender and social and economic influences, came into play. In the area there are well-developed institutional and community supports for sports such as soccer, rugby league and union,

Australian Rules Football and cricket, which often had strong links to local schools. On the other hand, for the young women, community sports and activities were either limited, or not easily accessed without a degree of family resources, which were often not available. School sport and physical education provided the main opportunities for organized physical activity. However, even in this context, being able to follow their interests was a much more chancy thing: electives were only available for some years; and the viability of sport teams relied on the interest of teachers and the motivation of other students. The following quote illustrates a common phenomenon for girls at all of the non-elite schools in this and other studies (e.g. Eime *et al.* 2008): that is, when it comes to organizing opportunities for physical activity, opportunities are often transitory and their existence relies on friendships and personal connections rather than institutional structures. What this suggests is that the physical activity identities of the young women from the government schools were formed in less structured contexts, compared to the physical activity identities of the students from the elite schools or many of the male students at the non-elite schools.

> I used to play softball, last season 'cause this season we couldn't get a team together or a coach to coach us. It was outside of school, and this year, I played for the school for softball at State. We used to have like, sport every Wednesday and a group of my friends, about 10 of us, we'd go play softball and we got through the whole season undefeated, first in the whole, in the whole thing. So we were pretty happy because some of them didn't even know how to play the game and we'd go just do this, I'll tell you what to do.
>
> (Felicia, interview Year 11 2000)

Like their counterparts at Sunnydale, for the young women at Greenvalley High limited community resources meant that school sport and physical education were their main sources of physical activity participation (see also Eime *et al.* 2008). For the boys from this school, however, farm work, BMX and functional physical activity were more likely to be part of their lives (see Chapter 1; Lee 2003).

Physical activity identities in the contexts of the government schools on the urban fringe and in the semi-rural area were more diverse and their expression – that is, choices of physical activity – more likely to be defined by gender, ethnicity and limited social and economic resources. As will be demonstrated later, when these young people left school, their choices and chances of physical activity participation were impacted by other priorities (and other identities) and also by the degree to which these choices were associated with 'pleasure' in busy lives, where time not dedicated to work or study was to be treasured.

Physical activity identities beyond school

For all of the young people managing priorities was intensified after leaving school; their lives illustrate the complex and complicated spaces that young people are negotiating as they endeavour to 'make' a life for themselves. Reading through the transcripts of all of the young people, we were struck by how busy their lives were. Having said this, their lives, as illustrated by some of the following quotes, took very different forms, which, in turn, had consequences for what physical activity meant to them, and the place or not it had in their lives.

For many of the young people from Sunnydale, and the elite schools (less so for Seachrist), the institutionalized context of school organized not only their time but their physical activity. When these organizing structures were removed, the young people were in a position where participation like other aspects of their life became a matter of individual responsibility. Their ongoing participation was contingent on a number of things: opportunities and access continued to be important, but the extent to which the notion of being physically active had become interpellated into the young person's notion of 'self', and the extent to which it had become included in the priority process around daily life, was also a major influence. It is not surprising then that, following the earlier discussions, the degree to which the young people participated in physical activity and the form that this took varied on class and gender lines.

The young women who had attended the elite girls school and who had subscribed to the school ethos around physical activity (all of the young women in the study except for Tomiko who had never been very interested in physical activity and for whom music had been more important), actively sought out new forms of physical activity that suited their busy lives beyond school. They explained these choices in terms of the balance it brought to their busy lives so that they could be more productive (at study or work). For these young women, physical activity was so embedded in their identities, almost like a visceral need. Physical activity was talked about as providing an essential 'balance' to the stresses of study and then work; it allowed them to juggle study, work and relationships and still maintain their health and well-being. Kim, for example, despite managing two university degrees, extracurricular activities that fitted with her social justice agenda, and catching up with friends and family, played and trained at least twice a week for competitive frisbee. Kim managed all of this by using her university as a one-stop shop for managing study, physical activity, socializing and work.

In a similar way Melinda used her physical activity to provide her with many of the necessities for a balanced life while at the same time assisting her with her career. Like most of the young women interviewed from the elite school, she had a clear idea about where she wanted to go with her life, even in general terms, and what she needed to do to get there. This included personal goals around exercise and body shape and weight. In school she cycled and jogged to achieve her 'exercise goals'; after school she took up dragon boat racing to help build the skills she perceived she needed for her future.

> Well I did it for dragon boating a little bit because I wanted dragon boating, because I knew dragon boating could give me things for my career, like it could give me leadership through captaincy and give me organizational skills and I wanted to give something back to the team because I knew that we had so much more potential and it just wasn't organized. So by putting time and effort into that I think it helped me form my career a bit more.
>
> (Melinda, interview 2006)

Building skills was clearly not the only reason that Melinda took up dragon boat racing, but in a very busy life it allowed her to manage the expectations she has about being social (friends and team) and maintaining her exercise, as well as building her career.

The young men from the elite school found it initially a bit of a struggle to adapt to a life where sport was no longer fully organized for them, but soon found new forms of organization via university or social networks. The young men we interviewed replaced school sport with more social sport, going to the gym and/or jogging or working out. They still talked about physical activity as though it were taken for granted as a part of 'a life', but now it had to be/could be more spontaneous and needed to be organized around their study, work and social lives. This took some getting used to. The following quote from Aaron is typical of the way they talked about their 'choices' about physical activity after leaving school. Eventually they were, however, all in social teams or jogging or spending time at the gym.

> It's a little different, you've got to sort of motivate yourself to do stuff; you don't have anyone sort of relying on you to be doing this work if you don't want to. I guess I sort of prefer the way that school was organized because then you always had things to do like to do with sport; you know it was a lot easier to get into back then.
>
> (Aaron, interview 2006)

As indicated earlier the physical activity identities of the young people from the government schools and Seachrist College were far more diverse and less likely to be so central to their sense of self. In other words physical activity was usually seen as a good thing (particularly in relation to health), but except for Karin none of the young women talked about a visceral need to be active; it became something optional and low in the priorities when other aspects of their lives took precedence. It also took on different meanings with new relationships and changing life circumstances. Felippe, for example, who had shown little interest in physical activity at school or immediately after, by his last interview, having left university to focus on his job, had also begun to work out regularly with his brother every morning because he wanted to build some muscle and put on weight.

> Yes it is, I feel healthy. For a little while I was taking it very seriously, like I'd be walking five days a week as well, just to get some exercise because I don't really exercise. I was walking a little bit and then I was doing the weights as well. But I realized with the walking I was losing a lot of weight and so I thought I've got to stop doing it because I want to gain weight.
>
> (Filippe, interview 2006)

Immediately after leaving school many of the young people from the government and coast schools were trying to combine part-time study and part-time or full-time work. The work was still often poorly paid and involved shifts at night and on the weekend. The little time and energy left was often spent socializing/clubbing with friends or partners. For someone like Rusty, an ex-Seachrist student, this was not too onerous because he lived at home and surfing could be fitted in anytime around commuting to Sydney for study, working as a bar manager and socializing. Tamara, on the other hand, who had been so active during her school years, was more interested in partying, working hard and studying for a childcare diploma. Eve, who in the 2002 interview was still playing hockey after years of representing at school because it would 'feel weird not to', stopped in 2004 because she worked on Saturdays. By 2005 she had begun going to the gym with her boyfriend to fit activity around full-time work. In 2007, she was engaged, working long hours and because of the long hours and an injury stopped going to the gym, but had bought a WiFi game for exercise. Eve, Chrissie and Tamara used the gym too because it helped them keep fit and could be fit flexibly into their busy lives (see Chapter 4).

For Karin, Felicia, Cassie and Sharon, there was a stronger sense of a struggle around physical activity, often talked about as something they would like to do but which they found extremely difficult to fit into their lives. This sense of other priorities interfering with their choice to do some form of physical activity increased over the three years of interviews following school, as their lives became more complicated by health issues, relationships and the continual need to find employment; for some it was complicated by the responsibilities of parenthood or for elderly members of the family. For example, in the following quote Felicia nostalgically compares a time (at school) when physical activity was not a choice, with her life as the mother of two young boys. Despite her description of 'home' as a place where nothing is compulsory, what she seems to mean is that 'home' is a place where it is impossible to plan for anything on a regular basis because the everyday life of a mother with two children whose partner works two jobs has little room for time out to go to the park on a regular and predictable basis.

> Yes and then once I left [school] I stopped [playing softball] completely, mostly because your mind is concentrating on what you want to do and you don't have time to exercise. In school you've got the teachers and it is compulsory and then you have a choice whether you want to compete or not. Whereas at home every day nothing is compulsory and you can do what you want when you want. . . . So when you've got swimming carnivals and sport on specific day it is a thing you have to do. Whereas at home if you've got two kids and Wednesday is sport day you don't find many households who are going to go by that rule. Parents say 'every Thursday we'll go to the park' that will encourage kids to do more exercise. But very rarely you'll find someone that does that.
>
> (Felicia, interview 2005)

For Karin who had been a very keen hockey player at school and who had described physical activity in earlier interviews as absolutely necessary for maintaining her weight and feeling fine about her body, this priority had been replaced (not easily) with the need to work and earn money for her future security. Her almost compulsive need to exercise had been (at least for the time being) replaced by the demands of her work, which, in her final interviews, she described as deeply satisfying. She was winning awards for her work as a pastry chef; and she saw her success as allowing her to realize her dream of setting up a business and buying a house in Queensland, with her partner. As she points out in her last interview, there was little time for any leisure in her life:

> I want to achieve a lot with my career and work wise so I know I have to put in the hours but then I feel like I'm missing out on the rest; like the social life, you know, just going for a bike ride, taking the kayak out, motorbike. And when you do think alright I've got the time to do it you are just so worn out that you just don't want to do it. It's too much effort. So you just feel tired all the time.

> (Karin, interview 2006)

Karin missed physical activity because it has in the past afforded her a great deal of pleasure. She can imagine a time when it will be restored to her.

For the young women from the semi-rural area, Sharon and Cassie, travelling and working long hours, spending time with family and when possible having some time to do the things they liked doing (gave them some pleasure) took priority over physical activity. For example Sharon, who, while at school played competitive touch football and netball (until her knees prevented her), was, in her last interview, working long hours managing a bottle shop, studying to get work in security and living at home with her mum. Pleasure lay with a good movie in bed or if she could afford it going to the Gold Coast with friends.

> Weekends I don't do many things because I work Tuesday through to Saturday so I can't really go out Friday night because Saturday is such a big day at work and then Saturday night I'm just exhausted from the week. I just want to curl up in bed with a movie if I'm lucky.

And later in the interview when asked: 'What kind of things would make you happy?'

> Being able to do stuff on my days off because I have the money to do it. Like just go to the [Gold] Coast for a night would be good, just go to the beach. I can't even go for a day trip because it's extra fuel and it's money that I don't have. I don't know, just things like that, catching up with friends.

Inflexible and long work hours also made it difficult to take up physical activities that did not fit with her roster.

Int: So apart from work, which seems to take up the majority of your time, are you doing anything else, any physical activity or leisure stuff?

Sharon: I just bought a camera so I want to get into Photography on my days off. So I'll actually have a hobby. So I'll feel like I'm working for something.

And I did start doing some kickboxing but then my roster changed so I couldn't do it anymore.

Int: Did you go somewhere and do that?

Sharon: Yes, that's just at [place] about five, ten minutes away from my place. So it was good, nice and convenient and easy.

(Sharon, interview 2006)

Cassie who by her own description has never enjoyed sport very much was also working long hours in a childcare centre with children with special needs, planning for her marriage, living with her grandmother and taking her mother shopping in her spare time. In this quote what is particularly interesting, besides the demands of travelling and work, is how she seems to feel the need to explain to the interviewer that she is doing *some* exercise; that is, heavy physical work and walking to work gets conceptualized as a 'good thing' because it provides some 'exercise'.

Well generally on the weekends I usually work from Monday until Saturday. So I work six days. And then the Sunday I'll spend at home with my grandmother and we'll just go out and do the shopping or do things like that. I don't really, because I work in Brisbane I'm having to, I get up early, I go to work and then I come back and by the time I get back it's relatively late and I'm pretty tired. So I'll have dinner and sit down and watch TV for a little bit and then go to bed.

And later in the same interview

Work is really good because I walk. Some days I'll walk home from the train station or I'll walk to the train station and then I walk from the train station to work and I'm doing all the heavy lifting like loading and unloading linen and then pushing them up on to each of the wards.

(Cassie, interview 2006)

Conclusion

For most of the young people in the *Life Activity Project* whom we were able to interview after leaving school, school was one of the major (re)sources for physical activity in their lives. For the coast young people, and particularly the male students, the beach and the surf provided other resources. The kinds of physical activity identities that the young people developed, however, differed particularly in relation to the social class effects of the elite boys and girls schools, and the value placed by the schools and then the young people, on physical activity as an essential part of a 'balanced life'. When the organizing structure for physical activity (through school) was removed, physical activity did not disappear from the young people's lives, but was (like all other aspects of life) largely translated into an individual responsibility.

For all the young people in the study, managing competing priorities was intensified after school – all struggled to negotiate a combination of work/study/social life/relationships/family. Their 'choices' around physical activity were made in this context *and* in relation to their physical activity identities. In addition, for some, the desire to be active in the ways they enjoyed could not be realized because of non-negotiable factors such as cost of participation and the priority of family responsibilities. The interplay of physical activity identities formed in the school years, the competing priorities in young people's lives, and social and cultural constraints need to be recognized in the commentary on young people's declining rates of physical activity. Discourses of blame are not productive in assisting young people. Rather community strategies to reduce costs and to make relevant forms of physical activity more accessible through free access to gyms and good quality childcare would make a difference for at least some of the young people in our study and young people in similar situations. School experiences that help to shape positive physical activity identities would also be helpful.

References

Abbott-Chapman, J. (2000) 'Time out spaced out: young people making meaning', *Youth Studies Australia*, 19(1): 21–25.

Ball, S. J., Macquire, M. and Macrae, S. (2000) *Choice, Pathways and Transitions Post-16: new youth, new economies in the global city*, London: Routledge/Falmer.

Beck, U. and Beck-Gernsheim, E. (2002) *Individualization*, London: Sage.

Eime, R. M., Payne, W. R., Casey, M. M. and Harvey, J. T. (2008) 'Transition in participation in sport and unstructured physical activity for rural living adolescent girls', *Health Education Research*, doi:10.1093/her/cyn060 (accessed 24 January 2010).

Fitzclarence, L. (2004) 'Bodies, bombs and belief systems: sport, lifestyle construction and education in dangerous times', *Sport, Education and Society*, 9(2): 253–67.

Gyurcsik, N., Bray, S. and Brittain, D. (2004) 'Coping with barriers to vigorous physical activity during transition to university', *Family and Community Health*, 27(2): 130–42.

Lee, J. (2003) 'The place and meaning of physical activity, physical education, and physical culture in the lives of young people living in rural Queensland', *Education in Rural Australia*, 13(2): 27–46.

Leslie, E., Fotheringham, M. J., Owen, N. and Bauman, A. (2001) 'Age-related differences in physical activity levels of young adults', *Medicine and Science in Sports and Exercise*, 33(2): 255–58.

Rees, G., Fevre, R., Furlong, J. and Gorard, S. (1997) 'History, place and the learning society: towards a sociology of lifetime learning', *Journal of Education Policy*, 12(6): 485–97.

Rose, G. (1992) *The Strategy of Preventive Medicine*, Oxford: Oxford University Press.

Sallis, J., Prochaska, J. and Taylor. W. (2000) 'A review of correlates of physical activity of children and adolescents', *Medicine and Science in Sports and Exercise*, 32(5): 963–75.

Slee, R. (2000) 'Preface', in S. J. Ball, M. Macquire, and S. Macrae (eds) *Choice, Pathways and Transitions Post-16: new youth, new economies in the global city*, London: Routledge/Falmer.

White, R. and Wyn, J. (2004) *Youth and Society: exploring the social dynamics of youth experience*, Melbourne: Oxford University Press.

Wright, J. and O'Flynn, G. (2007) 'Social class, femininity and school sport', in J. McLeod and A. Allard (eds) *Learning from the Margins: young women, social exclusion and education*, London and New York: Routledge.

Wright, J., O'Flynn, G. and Macdonald, D. (2006) 'Being fit and looking healthy: young women's and men's constructions of health and fitness', *Sex Roles – A Journal of Research*, 54(9–10): 707–16.

Wyn, J. and Dwyer, P. (1999) 'New directions in research on youth in transition', *Journal of Youth Studies*, 2(1): 5–21.

Wyn, J. and Woodman, D. (2006) 'Generation, youth and social change in Australia', *Journal of Youth Studies*, 9(5): 495–514.

11 The *Life Activity Project* in the American inner-city

Multi-ethnic young people's engagements with health discourses

Matthew Atencio

Introduction

As noted by Crawford in 1980, 'health' has become 'a national preoccupation' and is symbolic of 'a metaphor for all that is good in life' (p. 365). In contemporary times, this notion of the 'good life' is underpinned by the neo-liberal assumption that being 'healthy' is part of a moral and productive life. From this perspective, the term 'healthism' has come to represent the dominant health ideologies which hold individuals responsible for avoiding 'lazy or poor personal habits' related to exercise and eating, and for making the choice to take up 'a more health-promoting lifestyle' (Crawford 1980: 368) in order to attain 'healthy' selves and bodies.

Health 'experts' and proponents play a key role in (re)producing this healthism discourse. They argue that individuals can prevent 'lifestyle diseases' by avoiding risky lifestyle practices and taking up prescribed healthy eating and exercise practices. In the context of what has been termed an 'obesity epidemic' (Gard and Wright 2005), these health practices are also seen as a means of counteracting the effects of overeating, poor eating choices and sedentary lifestyles. O'Flynn (2004: 7) suggests that moralistic and individualistic health discourses operate in tandem with broader 'risk' discourses 'to create a context of fear and anxiety' in western societies. Because the healthism discourse directly impacts upon young people's sense of self, there is a need to understand the ways these health 'truths' impact upon young people's 'desires, actions and beliefs' (Fullagar 2003: 48).

Arguably, members of the 'white' middle class most often support and benefit from prevailing constructions of health in western societies (Crawford 1980; Edgley and Brissett 1990). Azzarito (2009: 184) suggests that dominant notions of health are 'colour blind' and 'monocultural' (e.g. representing whiteness); she argues that dominant 'fitness and health crusades in school physical education panopticize non-whites, the populations most at risk for fatness, as visibly different, abnormal, unhealthy and lazy'. She reminds us that health discourses are mediated by young people's personal and cultural histories that are racial and ethnic in nature.

While Azzarito's work describes the key health discourses that influence minority-ethnic young people's lives, Rail (2009) more closely examines how these individuals construct identities relative to these health discourses. In her study of multi-ethnic Canadian youths, Rail describes the complex and fluid process by which health discourses are negotiated:

> Consider, for example, a young Somali-Canadian participant who had to nego-tiate a position within a discourse dominant in her Black, Muslim, Somali-Canadian community as well as a position within a discourse dominant among her mostly white, Christian, Euro-Canadian schoolmates. In general, partici-pants could be seen as moving in and out of their various subject positions with considerable ease. In discussing health, they were generally involved in dis-cursive practices that produced gender, race, or dis/ability as a reiteration of hegemonic norms, yet their performative acts also transpired fluidity and the possibility of interpellation by alternative discourses.
>
> (Rail 2009: 152)

From this perspective, then, young people from minority-ethnic backgrounds engage with health discourses in fluid ways; that is, in various social contexts and by drawing upon a range of personal and cultural resources, their engagements come to reflect conformity and resistance.

It is from this perspective that I examine how young people from ethnic minority backgrounds in an inner-city neighbourhood in the United States engage with 'healthism' discourses and in doing so construct particular racial and gendered identities.

Methodology

In the *Life Activity Project*, the study that informs this chapter, eight young women and nine young men between the ages of 13 and 18 were recruited from an urban American neighbourhood (see Chapter 3 for more detail on the study). The partici-pants came from a range of minority-ethnic and immigrant backgrounds. Each par-ticipant[1] was asked questions about health, sport and physical activity during five to seven interviews. Like the other *Life Activity Project* studies, one of the thematic interviews investigated young people's meanings about health; these are the focus of this chapter. This involved asking young people what it meant to be 'healthy', what was required to live a 'healthy' life, and whether they found 'healthiness' to be a desirable state. During these interviews the young people were also shown examples of athletes and other physical activity participants in order to discuss their constructions of body image and eating/exercise practices. The young people were asked to describe: what they found to be unhealthy; what unhealthy people looked and acted like; whether or not they wanted to be unhealthy (as they understood the concept); and also, what their various sources of health information were. I asked the participants to rate themselves on a scale of 1–10 ('1' being the unhealthiest) to investigate the degree to which young people felt that they were healthy or unhealthy and to prompt discussions about why this might be so. In order to closely consider the young people's health engagements, in this chapter I only highlight commentary from three young men (John, Adam and Neal) and four young women (Sara, Sharon, Maureen and Monet) from the study.

Maureen moved to the United States from Haiti when she was 11 years old. She lived with an older sister in a housing estate that was known for drug dealing and criminal activities. Maureen participated in the high school dance team, and she also danced in clubs or house parties. She ran track for the team, although she quit because she said that she did not get along with her coaches. When asked to rate her own health on a scale of 1–10, with '10' being the highest, Maureen described herself as a 'five'. She explained this as being because: 'I might be healthy, but not as healthy, as everyone should be, because I just don't do things, so I don't stay healthy, and that's my reason'.

Sarah described herself as a Hispanic/French-Canadian, and she came from a middle-class neighbourhood on the periphery of the research site. Sarah participated in the local high school dance classes and recitals until she injured her back during her third year. She subsequently worked as a backstage assistant for recitals and performances. She also played volleyball and walked regularly. Sarah had a very thin and toned body. Sarah rated herself as 'five or six' because she would sometimes eat things that she considered 'unhealthy'; however, she also said that eating 'unhealthy' foods once in a while was 'fun'.

Sharon and Monet were sisters who identified themselves as Cherokee (Native American)/African American/white. Their single mother worked at a local shipping company and, as such, they were relatively more financially secure than some of the other young women in the study, who were primarily from impoverished backgrounds. At the high school, Sharon participated in African and hip hop dance classes in the morning, and took ballet and more advanced African classes in the afternoon. After school she participated in the school performance group and she also danced regularly in a local African dance festival. Her younger sister Monet attended a Catholic high school and was involved in dance and basketball. When asked to rate themselves, Monet considered herself to be an 'eight', while Sharon said she was a 'six-point-five'. Monet described herself as a 'fitness freak' and said she would do sit-ups before going to bed. Sharon explained her 'six-point-five' as being because she walked and danced, but sometimes ate junk food.

There was far less social class differentiation amongst the young men. These African American young men came from impoverished sections of the city, and had come to consider basketball as the means to personal success. Adam's father mentored youth in a local community centre while his mother worked as a middle-school teacher. Adam played point guard for the high school basketball team, which often contended for the state championship. Adam said that he was a '10' because: 'I'm really healthy, I mean I workout all the time, but it's not to a point that I run around the track all the time, I run around the basketball court'.

Neal's parents were divorced and he moved back and forth between his father's and mother's houses. Neal played basketball with Adam in the parks, and also on the high school and elite travelling teams. Like Adam, Neal considered basketball to be a 'tool' to escape a life surrounded by poverty and crime; he often referred to extended family members and peers who had become 'caught up' in drugs or gangs. Neal said that he was an 'eight' because, 'I'll stay away from drugs' and also because he ate the 'right stuff' and kept his body 'in shape'.

John lived with his mother, stepfather and younger brother. John's older brother was a former football star whose playing career was eventually curtailed because he became involved in gangs and crime and was subsequently incarcerated. John was physically much shorter than Adam and Neal and had a stockier body build. He did not try out or play for the high school basketball team and played reserve team grid-iron football. John ranked himself as a 'six', because he could 'still run fast and lift weights'. He said that could 'carry his weight' in sport, which was important, since he was 'overweight kinda'.

'Like a fat person sitting on the couch': young people's constructions of healthy and unhealthy practices

When initially asked to discuss what it meant to be healthy, the young people consistently described healthiness in terms of eating and exercising properly. This understanding of health as related to eating and exercise practices became more evident when questions around health were framed in the negative, as in, 'what does it mean to be unhealthy?' The young people linked unhealthiness with moral laxity and associated this state with a range of other undesirable practices (e.g. eating 'bad' foods and being lazy). Often, it was assumed that eating 'badly' was linked to getting overweight. According to all of the young people, a person's ability to adhere to healthy practices was manifested in their bodily appearance. Sarah's quote exemplifies this position:

Int: How can you tell if someone is healthy? How can you tell that they are healthy?

Sarah: Probably just by physical appearance, I mean people might actually be healthy, and not look too healthy, but to me, if I see someone who is not really overweight, I guess, then I'm like well they probably know what they're doing, right or wrong.

(Sarah, interview 2002)

The ways in which the young people read unhealthiness from the appearance of the body becomes further evident in the following exchange with Sharon and Monet:

Int: What do you think a 'one' would be like?

Sharon: Probably eat anything and everything and not just that, but would be a couch potato, even if you do eat a lot, if you work out occasionally, that will move you down the scale [and improve your health] . . .

Int: Monet, what do you think?

Monet: Yeah, like a fat person sitting on the couch, eating a whole bag of chips, not walking anywhere, or going anywhere, never does anything.

(Sharon and Monet, interview 2002)

Regardless of sport and dance background, both young men and young women all seemed to believe that bodies could be read for their healthiness or unhealthiness; appearance was linked with moral judgements about particular behaviours – the 'couch potato' or 'fat person sitting on the couch' was the primary signifier of unhealthiness.

Taken together, the young people's initial comments suggest that they 'bought into' the healthism discourse, whereby knowledge and characteristics associated with 'healthiness' and 'unhealthiness' are evidenced by the size, shape and exercise capacity of the body. In this way they were very similar to the responses reported by young [white] people in other studies (Burrows and Wright 2004; Rail 2009). I now turn to illustrate how later interview exchanges more explicitly illustrate the ways discourses around health intersected with broader cultural discourses of race, ethnicity, culture and gender, and were taken up differently by the young people, and particularly the young women as compared to the young men.

'You gotta be good, or you won't win it': young men's constructions of health and bodies through sport

Neil, Adam and John's responses to questions about health suggested that health for them was primarily about keeping their bodies strong for successful performance in their particular sports. For example, this is evident in the following quote from John:

Int: Is being healthy something that um, you think about or is a part of your life? And if it is, in what ways is it?

John: Yeah, I try to eat like, some fruit, sometimes, like four days out of the week. Try to pump some iron five times a week. [It's] Important to me to lift weights.

Int: How come?

John: I'm tryin' to go to the league.

Int: Try to go to which league?

John: The NFL [National Football League].

(John, interview 2003)

The young men linked health with adherence to specified eating and exercise practices – being healthy involved eating and drinking properly and adhering to a physically intensive exercise regimen. John summed up this approach to health with the formula, 'pump weights, eat right'. As mentioned previously, the young men and women felt that adherence to health practices could be read off the body because these practices allowed one to 'stay in shape'. Yet, for the young men in particular, being 'in shape' usually implied having a 'nice body' or the 'right look' – usually a muscular or athletic body that was devoid of excess fat and would help the person perform better in his particular sport. Even if someone was considered to be overweight, the young men felt that as long as the person could 'carry their weight', usually in the context of a sport contest, then this person was still healthy. Across all the interviews, the young men did not mention that 'fat' or 'overweight' people were unattractive in appearance or were health risks. For them, their moral evaluation of 'fat' and 'overweight' people was linked with the belief that these individuals could not play basketball or football at a high standard. John, Adam and Neal, who wanted to use sport as a means of getting university athletic scholarships, did not only surveil and regulate their own bodies, but also monitored the bodies, and eating and exercise practices, of their peers. For both Neal and Adam, those who did not make the 'correct' choices around dominant health knowledges and practices were 'letting the team down' because they played 'slow'.

Notions of individual choice and self-improvement that are associated with health dovetailed with competitive sport discourses and spoke powerfully to these young men. Kirk (2004: 129) argues that in a disciplinary society, the practices associated with sport, 'fitness' and the 'new dietary regimes' work closely together in order to produce very similar kinds of idealized bodies. While the young men were subject to the technologies of power that rendered their bodies docile through sport training, the young men also *chose* to work on their selves and bodies by taking up these disciplinary practices. I argue that young men such as Adam, John and Neal actively came to reflect upon and make choices, usually in assimilationist ways, in relation to these intersecting health and sport discourses. Adam, John and Neal actively participated in the construction of an embodied healthy self that was linked to the goal of sport success. This goal was hugely important for them in the context of impoverished urban neighbourhoods where community leaders and corporations such as Nike promoted 'self-empowerment through sport' ideals.

Young women's constructions of 'overweight' and 'fat' bodies

Further into their interviews, the young women talked at greater length about the issue of being 'bigger' or even 'fat'. While Maureen was quite vehement about her disdain for 'fat' people, Sharon, Monet and Sarah, who came from more middle-class backgrounds and largely participated in activities such as dance and cheerleading, seemed to be less negative in their judgements. Maureen's descriptions, in particular, suggest that she constructed her sense of self through the constitution of an 'abject' 'fat' Other (Grosz 1994; Kristeva 1982). Young (1990: 143) describes 'abjection' as 'the feeling of loathing and disgust the subject has in encountering certain matter, images, and fantasies – the horrible, to which it can only respond with aversion, with nausea and distraction'. Employing this concept of abjection, Braziel and Lebesco (2001: 130) have suggested that 'fat' women's bodies have become 'synonymous with the horrible, or deadly aspects of embodiment'.

In the following exchange, Maureen describes how, for her, 'overweight' people were 'nasty':

Int: What would a 'one' be like on the scale, say 'one' being unhealthiest, and, yeah, would you want to be a 'one'?

Maureen: No, I wouldn't want to be a 'one', because I wouldn't want to be an overweight person, because you know how people just overweight, they don't care, they eat anything, and they eat fast food, and they usually don't care how their body looks like, that's just nasty.

(Maureen, interview 2003)

Previous to this exchange, Maureen had talked about how her Haitian friend, Darlene (who was also in the study), was 'really, really lazy' because she did not eat right and failed to train hard for track; Maureen described how Darlene became slower and eventually stopped running and how she did not 'respect that'. In this instance, Maureen's comments reflect the sport performance discourse evident in the young men's talk about health. For them, it was acceptable to be larger but only if this did not preclude the person from performing in sport; one should be able to 'carry his weight'. Maureen said that she was very comfortable weighing 125 pounds and talked about how she gained immense pleasure through her body by sprinting competitively and dancing (indeed, she enjoyed sensual 'freak' dancing in clubs and at house parties). From this position, then, Maureen came to understand and indeed appreciate her embodied self relative to her portrayal of 'fat' people who were 'disgusting' and 'lazy'.

Despite her highly toned and very trim body, Sarah commented that she did not think or talk about health very much, unless 'like if something has a lot of fat':

Int: Go ahead, go ahead and explore [what an unhealthy person looks like] a bit more.

Sarah: I don't know [laughs] kind of like . . . I don't know . . . just kind of . . . I don't know, people in my sense who would be bigger . . . I don't know, it's terrible! [laughs].

Int: It's fine, you can say what you want to.

Sarah: I don't know, I guess a little bigger, like maybe stomach hangs over their pants or their arms are really big, and . . . I don't know . . . [laughs] I just feel bad, picking some poor person apart! I don't know, I think that's kind of my idea, of someone who isn't exactly fit.

(Sarah, interview 2003)

While Sarah seems to mock overweight people in the previous exchange, in comparison to Maureen she seemed more sympathetic. Like Maureen, Sarah said she was content with her body size and unconcerned about gaining weight: 'I have a high metabolism and I'm not like, "Oh if eat all this, am I going to gain weight?"' Sharon also did not talk about fat people in the same derogatory way as Maureen. For example, she had herself experienced othering by her dance instructors who expected her to lose weight and 'work' on her body in order to be thin. She described how AfricanAmerican young women, such as herself, in the dance classes at the high school often experienced discrimination because of their 'overweight' bodies. Sarah confirmed this, describing how 'bigger' African American young women tended to be marginalized in comparison to the thin 'white girls'. It is likely then that these two young women's involvement in school dance came to inform their opinion about and sensitivity to being 'larger'.

Young women's resistance to 'healthy' eating and exercise practices

I now further describe how some of the young women, in particular, more directly resisted healthist directives and notions of bodily perfection in order to constitute their embodied subjectivities. As noted previously, the young men were primarily concerned with constituting embodied selves through highly disciplinary eating and exercise practices, in order to achieve success in sport. In comparison, some of the young women's comments, later in the health interview, indicated that they actively contested the dominant dieting and exercise practices associated with self-control of the body.

In particular, the young women from African American and black Haitian backgrounds discussed eating to achieve bodily pleasure by consuming foods that health advocates would consider 'unhealthy'. Maureen, despite her strong views about 'fat' being disgusting, provided many statements indicative of this attitude. For example in the following exchange, she describes how she wants to eat 'everything' in order to feel 'lazy' and 'full'. Prior to the following quote, Maureen was describing how her friend Mandy was dieting because she wanted to lose weight. Maureen then commented that she did not feel compelled to adopt such dieting practices:

Maureen: The only thing she [her friend Mandy] talks about health is eating healthy and not eating a lot of junk food, like keeping off the ice cream, just stay off that, and drink water.
Int: And what do you think about that?
Maureen: [Laughs] Well, I don't think there's any problem . . . like I said, I eat everything.

And later in the interview:

Int: How do you feel when you eat, say, burgers, ribs and chicken, and things like that?
Maureen: How do I feel? After eating it, I feel lazy, I'll be so full.
Int: Do you feel like you're still being healthy, or unhealthy?
Maureen: I don't feel bad [laughs] I really don't think about that, now that you brought that up, I really don't think about it.
Int: But physically you feel lazy or mentally you feel lazy?
Maureen: I feel lazy, like my whole body feels lazy, when you feel lazy you just can't do anything else and you just sit and can't move.
Int: Is that a good feeling?
Maureen: [Laughs] Uh huh, it's bad but then again it's good . . . because people can sit somewhere and it feels good not to move, I don't know why, but that's just how it is with me.

(Maureen, interview 2003)

When Maureen discussed eating, she dismissed the need to eat in accordance with the health knowledge that was given to her by her sport coaches. While she 'knew' that she was supposed to eat healthy, she chose to act differently. Maureen said that she did not feel guilty or 'bad' about the way she ate – even though she noted that she was supposed to ('it's bad'); eating tasty foods and not being able to move were very pleasurable embodied experiences for her. By refusing and indeed subverting the coaches' advice, Maureen constituted a particular relation to her self (Maureen makes a very strong claim to *not* doing anything that her coaches considered to be healthy). As she says, 'That's just me'. I earlier highlighted how Maureen negatively portrayed 'fat' people in abject ways. It seems for Maureen eating greasy and rich foods was acceptable as long as a person did not gain weight and become 'fat'. This meant constantly exercising, which she did in copious amounts through club dancing and running competitively. At the same time, she did not feel compelled to eat according to her coaches' advice because she did not gain weight and performed well on a regular basis.

Sharon also resisted health advice given to her by her dance teachers who wanted her to lose weight and work on her body:

> I had to struggle with, even with some of the teachers, you know, telling me that I needed to lose a little weight for this or I need to work on, just work on my body in general. I mean it wasn't a big deal with me because I already had the self-confidence and it didn't affect me.
>
> (Sharon, interview 2004)

Sharon also made reference to the 'skinny white girls' whom she encountered daily in her high school dance classes. She described these dancers as having 'no meat on their bones, just skinny for no reason'. By positioning these 'skinny white girls' as the abject 'Other', Sharon came to claim a sense of self linked with 'black' culture. She went on to describe how 'blacks' were more accepting of eating seemingly 'unhealthy' foods and having larger bodies. Sharon also commented that she enjoyed dancing with other 'black' people in her Kwanzaa[2] and African dance groups, where the 'rhythm' and the 'beat' were most important, rather than being 'thin' and worrying about 'losing weight'. She made fun of how the 'white' dancers would go to fast food restaurants and order hamburgers with no meat, cheese or mayonnaise. She claimed that these young women were too preoccupied with 'starving' and 'overworking' themselves in order to be 'skinny'. Like Maureen, Sharon felt confident about her body weight and thus did not see any reason to adhere to the disciplinary eating regimes advocated by her instructors.

Discussion

Azzarito (2009: 183) reminds us that health discourses are not racially neutral, as these discourses 'take place in a time of cultural hybridization'. From this perspective, I have illustrated above the multiple and contradictory ways in which 'health' was defined and practised by a group of minority-ethnic young people. Through my analysis, I argue that while minority-ethnic young people have been positioned as being 'problematic' and as 'health risks', studies have not paid enough attention to the nuanced and complex ways in which they take up and construct notions of health relative to intersecting discourses of the body, culture, race and ethnicity.

Disciplinary regimes associated with health, sport and physical activity came to significantly influence how the young people understood themselves and their peers as being either 'healthy' or 'unhealthy'. In their talk about health, the young people were able to (re)produce the dominant health imperatives which were linked to specific eating and exercising practices with a great deal of fluency. Based on their initial comments, I argue that the young people made moral judgements about health through a cyclical association of appearance, attitude and behaviour. In this way, the body was understood as portraying 'the virtuous health of the self' (Jutel 2005: 119), and one's ability to take care of their own body signified 'an exemplary technology of the self' (Leahy and Harrison 2004: 133). According to Foucault (1997), individuals have the freedom to transform themselves by taking up and negotiating particular discourses in order to become 'moral' subjects of their own actions. The psychic practices which lead to the constitution of an 'ethical' self are considered the 'technologies of the self'. As noted by Wright *et al.* (2006: 707), this concept is helpful to understand the multiple and complex ways that young women 'take up, negotiate, and resist the imperatives of the health and fitness discourses'. Following on this understanding of self-governing practices, it is possible to understand how and why minority-ethnic young people came to recognize and invest in particular health practices in order to constitute specific embodied subjectivities.

The young men and women involved in high performance sport often took up and reproduced a disciplinary approach to health, involving heavy regulation of the body. The young men, in particular, felt that the body needed to be subjected to healthy exercise and eating regimes in order to be prepared for sport performance. Research indicates that young men take up distinctive bodily practices that have much more to do with becoming 'fit', strong and capable rather than maintaining slimness or one's appearance. Wright *et al.*'s (2006) study of young men and young women in Australian schools, for instance, concluded that the young men did not exercise to improve their appearance. The young men valued forms of fitness which would give them strength, skill, and power in the context of performance sport – these attributes were associated with the constitution of a hegemonic masculine identity. Because they were preoccupied with regulating and working on their bodies, the young men were precluded from thinking about or moving the body in non-instrumental ways. They did not consider 'other body-self relationships that lie outside those of a taken-for-granted association between masculinity and competent physicality' (Wright *et al.* 2006: 715).

Maureen, a young woman involved in sprinting, came to negotiate health discourses in similar ways to the young men. However, for Maureen, abjecting the 'fat' Other was one means by which she came to construct her sense of self. According to Young (1990:145), 'the subject reacts to this abject with loathing as the means of restoring the border separating self and other'. From this perspective, then, the practice of creating a 'disgusting, abject unhealthy other' (Leahy 2009: 179) came to underpin her embodied self-formation. Sarah's and Sharon's position on 'fat' had been shaped, on the other hand, by their witnessing of the othering of 'bigger' African American young women in the dance programme.

To complicate matters further, both Sharon and Maureen spoke about the pleasure derived from resisting the eating and training advice given to them by instructors and coaches. They seemed to 'refuse' (Wright *et al.* 2006) specific practices involving work and discipline, by drawing upon their minority-ethnic cultures and involvement in cultural dance. Sarah, who most easily fitted the white middle-class ideal because of her light-skinned and thin appearance, seemed to reflect a more normative approach to eating. In contrast, I argue that 'black' cultural influences linked with hip hop and African dancing were important to how Maureen and Sharon negotiated and understood health and unhealthiness in non-conformist ways.

All of the young people were recruited based on their involvement in some form of physical activity. The young people described in this chapter were athletic and participated at a high standard in sport and dance. The young men mostly replicated healthist discourses that involved investing in great amounts of work relative to eating, 'working out' and training. The comments from Sarah, Maureen and Sharon were more reflective and complex. However, 'the notion of resistance can only be carried so far' (Rail 2009: 150) since these young women came from relatively privileged positions afforded them through their athletic and strong bodies. The social capital provided to them by their sport or dance trained bodies meant that they could take up seemingly critical subject positions regarding health. They could be playful or even critical about 'bigger' or 'fat' people because they themselves were in no real danger of becoming overweight. Taken together, then, the comments from the young women, in particular, reflected how they took up and negotiated health practices in relation to their bodies, which had been honed through sport and dance participation. At the same time, they negotiated dominant health practices made available to them in relation to their unique social class and cultural backgrounds, leading to diverse and complex health experiences.

Notes

1 The names of all participants have been changed to protect their anonymity.
2 Kwanzaa is a non-denominational 'African American' holiday incorporating African culture and ancestry.

References

Azzarito, L. (2009) 'The rise of corporate curriculum: fatness, fitness, and whiteness', in J. Wright and V. Harwood (eds) *Biopolitics and the 'Obesity Epidemic': governing bodies*, London: Routledge.

Braziel, J. and Lebesco, K. (2001) *Bodies Out of Bounds: fatness and transgression*, Berkeley: University of California Press.

Burrows, L. and Wright, J. (2004) 'The good life: New Zealand children's perspectives on health', *Sport, Education and Society*, 9(2): 193–205.

Crawford, R. (1980) 'Healthism and the medicalization of everyday life', *International Journal of Health Services*, 10(3): 365–88.

Edgley, C. and Brissett, D. (1990) 'Health Nazis and the cult of the perfect body: some polemical observations', *Symbolic Interaction*, 13(2): 257–79.

Foucault, M. (1997) 'The ethics of the concern for self as a practice of freedom', in P. Rabinow (ed.) *Michel Foucault: ethics, subjectivity and truth. The essential works of Foucault*, vol. 1, New York: The New Press.

Fullagar, S. (2003) 'Governing women's active leisure: the gendered effects of calculative rationalities within Australian health policy', *Critical Public Health*, 13(1): 47–60.

Gard, M. and Wright, J. (2005) *The Obesity Epidemic*, New York: Routledge.

Grosz, E. (1994) *Volatile Bodies*, Bloomington, IN: Indiana University Press.

Jutel, A. (2005) 'Weighing health: the moral burden of obesity', *Social Semiotics*, 15(2): 113–25.

Kirk, D. (2004) 'Beyond the "academic" curriculum: the production and operation of biopower in the less-studied sites of schooling', in B. Baker and K. Heyning (eds) *Dangerous Coagulations? The uses of Foucault in the study of education*, New York: Peter Lang.

Kristeva, J. (1982) *Powers of Horror: an essay in abjection*, New York: Columbia University Press.

Leahy, D. (2009) 'Disgusting pedagogies', in J. Wright and V. Harwood (eds) *Biopolitics and the 'Obesity Epidemic': governing bodies*, London: Routledge.

Leahy, D. and Harrison, L. (2004) 'Health and physical education and the production of the "at risk" self', in J. Evans, B. Davies and J. Wright (eds) *Body, Knowledge and Control: studies in the sociology of physical education and health*, London and New York: Routledge.

O'Flynn, G. (2004) 'Young women's meanings of health and physical activity: the body, schooling, and the discursive constitution of gendered and classed subjectivities', Unpublished PhD dissertation, Wollongong, Australia: University of Wollongong Online. Available URL http://ro.uow.edu.au/theses/226/ (accessed 2 February 2010).

Rail, G. (2009) 'Canadian youth's discursive constructions of health in the context of obesity discourse', in J. Wright and V. Harwood (eds) *Biopolitics and the 'Obesity Epidemic': governing bodies*, London: Routledge.

Wright, J., O'Flynn, G. and Macdonald, D. (2006) 'Being fit and looking healthy: young women's and men's constructions of health and fitness', *Sex Roles*, 54(9–10): 707–16.

Young, I. M. (1990) *Justice and the Politics of Difference*, Princeton, NJ: Princeton University Press.

12 'Building castles in the sand'

Community, context and physical culture

Lisette Burrows

Introduction

As is the case in most western contexts, the notion that everyone everywhere (Gard 2004) is in the grip of an obesity epidemic has tremendous purchase in New Zealand (Burrows and Wright 2007). Unsurprisingly, children are pervasively represented as both a cause and as a potential solution to the problem (Burrows and Wright 2007) – a problem that at its most simplistic is framed in terms of an imbalance of inputs (food) and outputs (exercise) (Gard and Wright 2005; Wright and Dean 2007). In the inevitable search for causes or origins of the obesity problem, several lines of argument are repeatedly drawn on which contribute to a vision of the state of children and childhood, which in turn feeds into the *kinds* of solutions that are posed for young people. As Gard and Wright (2005) suggest, children are widely regarded as beings that spend far too much time watching television, playing computer games and engaging in other so-called sedentary pursuits. Various phenomena are blamed for this onset of sedentary behaviour, but chief among them are: first, the ready accessibility of new media technologies; second, the physical and social risks of unsupervised play; third, the assumed widespread parental practice of using televisions as 'baby-sitters'; and finally, the regularly rehearsed phrase, 'it's a different world we live in'. That is, an expanding population base; more awareness of 'stranger danger'; high density housing; a proliferation of cars; and a faster pace of life have replaced the 'good old days' where one could just release one's children out into the park to play (Hancox and Poulton 2006; Van den Bulck 2000). This kind of romanticizing of a past gone by is rehearsed frequently in popular media (Gard and Wright 2005) and is also a key argument employed in some geographical studies (Skelton and Valentine 1998; Valentine 1997, 2004) that have looked at the access young people have to spaces to be active.

Informing much of the commentary on unhealthy youth is a notion that not only have the social circumstances and environmental constraints of contemporary children's lives changed, but so have the very nature and constituents of childhood itself (Abbott-Chapman and Robertson 2008). Developmental psychologists talk of children 'growing up too soon' (Peterson 1996), cultural theorists point to the 'simulational world' within which children are presumed to exist (Featherstone 1991) while some youth researchers suggest that children 'are caught up, through long hours watching TV and videos, with the stories and myths (and values) of strangers' (Abbott-Chapman and Robertson 2002: 2). Still others write of young people being isolated from family and community and disconnected from life course pathways hitherto imagined (Martin 2002). What Laclau and Mouffe (1985) would call a 'collective imaginary' has emerged around the state of children and young people generally, and it would seem that health and/or physical activity markers have become crucial signifiers of this broader imaginary.

In this chapter I foreground the ways four 11-year-old New Zealand children engage in and think about physical activity in the context of their lives, in a small rural town called Wallacetown. I suggest that the universalistic accounts of children alluded to earlier fail to acknowledge the diverse contexts within which children engage in physical activity and that the solutions posed to a presumed nation-wide decline in youth physical activity are barely cognizant of the meanings children bring to their experiences of physical culture. I begin by briefly introducing the study context and methodology before teasing out some of the key meanings these children articulate for physical activity.

The research context

Wallacetown, in the South Island of New Zealand, was the site within which this study was undertaken. Wallacetown is a small rural town sandwiched between two large cities, each 50 km away. The major industry in Wallacetown is gold mining. The village centre houses two mini supermarkets, a garage, hair salons and a small selection of retail gift stores and takeaway food venues. Two public bars and a restaurant complement the basic services available in the town. Wallacetown Primary School, the context from which the participants were drawn, has a fluctuating student roll of 112 pupils. Nestled at the edge of the town, the school boasts large green fields, a substantial concreted courtyard for games and a play area equipped with the usual assortment of climbing bars and swings. It has a covered swimming pool, physical education storage shed and classrooms that were constructed 26 years ago.

This chapter draws on interviews conducted with four Year 6 children from Wallacetown school (i.e. 10–11 years old) – Kevin, Jack, Joanna and Melissa. The children were interviewed, using a semi-structured interview schedule, four times over the space of a year. Each interview was from 30 minutes to an hour in duration and the kinds of questions children were asked followed the LAP schedule (see Chapter 1). Interviews were transcribed verbatim with analysis focused on understanding the meanings the participants attributed to physical activity and on the nature of their physical activity experiences, both within and outside of schooling.

Meanings for physical activity

Physical activity = sport

MacDougall *et al.* (2004) and Pope (2006), researching Australian and New Zealand contexts respectively, are among those researchers who have pointed to the regular associations that young people make between the concept of physical activity and that of sport. Research on New Zealand tertiary physical education students' meanings for physical education points to the ways students regularly use the words 'sport' and 'physical education' interchangeably (Burrows 1999). Indeed, despite the best efforts of physical educators to emphasize the diverse learning activities their profession embraces, it would seem that many of those within – and most of those outside of – the profession still see sport and physical activity as synonymous (Stothart 1992). Given this, it was no surprise to see this sport/physical activity relationship reiterated by children in the current study.

Kevin, for example, is ten years old, lives with his parents, two brothers and a sister. He has moved towns three times and distinguishes the value of the towns he has lived in based on how many sporting options they afford. He clearly regards physical activity as 'sport' and further, 'sport' as formalized games with teams 'to join' and 'rules' to abide by. A youngster of few words his response to the interviewer's opening question was:

Int: What sort of physical activities were you involved in, beginning from when you were a very young child?
Kevin: Well [pause], I like to do sports.
Int: Yep. [pause] What kind of sports do you like to do?
Kevin: Rugby, tackle rugby, soccer, hockey, and that's all. And t-ball and softball.
Int: That's quite a lot. What about other than sport? Are there other physical activities apart from sport that you like to do?
Kevin: Um, no.

(Interview 1, Kevin)

When asked about his family's engagement in physical activities, Kevin referred to his brother and father as playing sports while his mother 'just stays around the house and tidies up' and his little sister plays games; 'she makes half of them up', he says. The hierarchy of value is clearly attributed to sports over 'games' and even, at this early age, the gendered dimensions of physical activity/leisure or at least, of Kevin's perceptions of them are beginning to be revealed.

Jack, a keen and successful motocross competitor, also clearly equated physical activity with sport. This was indicated in his response, 'Rugby, um, that's about it I think' when asked what types of physical activity he has been involved in. Interestingly, he did not refer to motocross riding as a 'sport' and hence it wasn't mentioned in his initial interview, despite his extensive and ongoing engagement in this pursuit. Joanna and Melissa too, from the outset, described sports as the predominant types of physical activity they have been involved in, listing tennis, netball, badminton, swimming, hockey and horse-riding as their physical activity repertoires.

Later interviews exploring the day-to-day lives of each of these young people revealed that sports were certainly *not* the only kinds of physical activities they engaged in. However, at a conceptual level, at least, the conflation of physical activity with sport endured throughout successive interviews with each of the children. As was the case in MacDougall *et al.*'s (2004) study, dancing and playing did not appear to count as physical activity, yet rugby and tennis certainly did. Given the explicit distinctions made between sport and physical activity in the context of New Zealand's school syllabus, *Health and Physical Education in the New Zealand Curriculum* (Ministry of Education, 1999),[1] this tendency to think and say 'sport' when asked about 'physical activity' is interesting. Further in light of the current pervasiveness of 'physical activity for health' messages both in and out of schools, we were a little surprised that children did not initially mention things like running, walking or other 'fitness-related' types of physical activity.

Descriptions of their involvement in sports ranged from detailed accounts of the logistics of participation (e.g. 'yeah – tennis is in the weekend and netball is through the school. Swimming is on Mondays and Thursdays and then badminton was just over at the hall'), through to descriptions of how it was they became interested in the sport in the first place and, on occasions, detailed reflections on what it is like to be involved in particular sports. For each of the children in our study, parental support and encouragement were acknowledged as key influences in their choice of sport. Melissa's mum was a tennis player, Kevin's dad played rugby, Jack's dad was a motocross rider and Joanna's mum was a regular swimmer. Each of the children played a range of sports including those their parents engaged in. They acknowledged that the cost of sport was a determining factor for how many different sports they could engage in and that their parents helped them by transporting them to games and practices and so on. Extended family, grandmas and nanas in particular, featured regularly in their descriptions of who and what encouraged their engagement in sport. Melissa's grandma takes her swimming every weekend, while Jack's nana supports him loudly from the sideline in his winter rugby games. Friends were also regarded as important influences on choices made between various sporting codes. When talking about *how* they decided to join particular sporting codes, for each of the children 'being with friends' was a key consideration. These findings are consistent with those derived from other sociological and psychological research around what motivates children's participation in sport (Chen 1996; Hills 2007; Smith 2003; Williams and Bedward 2002).

Kevin, a young Maori boy whose father is a policeman, seemed genuinely bemused by some of the questions we asked about his *own* participation in physical activity. The only time he got animated in the interviews was when talking about his family. He tended to answer 'what do *you* do' kinds of questions with '*we* do this …' answers, subverting the interviewer's intention to draw out his individual, personal proclivities. Indeed out of all of the participants, Kevin was the one who most consistently reflected on what different life phases (e.g. moving house, having a baby brother, etc.) for a family mean for what opportunities one might have for organized physical activity. Not that Kevin found it disturbing that he couldn't do certain things because of his family's shifting priorities. On the contrary, Kevin accepted these as part and parcel of family life – not a problem. For Kevin, physical activities, the ones he did himself *and* those that occurred in the context of his family life, were intimately tied to his relationship with family members. He played rugby because his brother and dad played. He enjoyed watching them play as much as doing it himself. When asked what felt good about going swimming, he said 'because it was nice to hang around with the family and do something together . . . it's just a fun activity'. This clear disposition towards engaging in family-based physical activities, coupled with a valuing of family per se is something regularly attributed to Maori in New Zealand (Bishop and Glynn 1999; Durie 1998; Jenkins and Ka'ai 1994). This is something that some commentators say is ignored by many contemporary health and/or physical activity initiatives that tend to draw from individualist rather than collective tenets (Sharples 2007).

Just playing

One of the key ways children talked about their physical activity (although they didn't call it this) was in the context of 'play'. Play was a descriptor used to refer both to activities happening in a school context and in their own time. An excerpt from Kevin's interview is illustrative of the regularity with which each of the children used the word 'play' to describe what they did in their daily lives.

Int: What do you do at lunchtime, if it's a fine day?

Kevin: I usually *play* outside. *Play* what my friends are playing. Usually they *play* ball tag. Or they just hang around, just *playing* and talking.

Int: What about after school? What happens after school?

Kevin: I *play* around. *Play* outside. Yesterday I was *playing* in the mud.

Int: What about in the holidays? What sorts of things do you like to do in the holidays?

Kevin: Sometimes we just stay at home, and *play* around, or go to the beach. Go over to a friend's house, or get someone over. Sometimes we go away and camp out. We'll go visit nana or – . [pause]

Int: When you go to the beach, what sorts of things do you do there?

Kevin: If it's a fine day, then dad usually gets some paua. And if it's not, then we just *play* around making castles, and building holes in the sand.

Int: What sort of things do you do while you are camping?

Kevin: We just *play* around. Have a walk round. Or stay in the tent and *play* games.

Int: What sort of physical activities do you do when you are camping?

Kevin: Well if we have a ball, we just *play* kicks. Or *play* a game of touch rugby.

(Interview 2, Kevin)

What interested us about the children's talk of play was that none of the activities they referred to in this way were mentioned in responses to questions that specifically asked them about their 'physical activity'. As the last line of Kevin's excerpt shows, when we introduced the word 'physical activity' into the question, the response shifted to a recognized sport, 'touch rugby'. This phenomenon reappeared in each of the interviews with the four participants. In their focus group interviews with young Australian children, MacDougall *et al.* (2004: 369) found that 'the terms "physical activity" and "exercise" had little meaning for children, who described them as terms adults use'. On the other hand, 'the meaning of "play" was immediately recognizable in all focus groups as different from sport, physical activity and fitness' (p. 379). For the participants in MacDougall *et al.*'s (2004: 380) study, descriptors associated with play included 'fun', 'spontaneity', 'interactions with friends', 'not too competitive' and 'not too aggressive', whereas those associated with physical activity were largely confined to things like 'running around', 'muscle building', 'weight-lifting' and engaging in various kinds of sports. In their view, the responses to the prompt 'play' also evoked a sense of neighbourhood and community that was not present when the children discussed 'physical activity' or 'sport' per se.

Asking each child to describe 'what they did last weekend' yielded information about their activities in the context within which they took place, often invoking detailed descriptions of their physical surrounds and the people with whom they shared these activities. We have included two children's descriptions of parts of their weekend here to provide a sense of the kind of lives all four children experience in Wallacetown, lives that no doubt would be unrecognizable to some of their big city counterparts.

Joanna describes her Saturday like this:

Joanna: We went rollerblading at their next-door neighbours' [her friends'] place. It's a big concrete – all their driveway is concrete, and there's quite a big hill and all that.
Int: Do you have your own roller blades?
Joanna: Yep.
Int: Oh good. So you take them around with you when you go to her house?
Joanna: Yeah. And, with the bikes – I had to borrow her big sister's. And my friend's got three other sisters. Two little ones and one big one. And we went for a walk down to a farm. We saw the baby turkeys. And the chickens and all that . . . Yep. And in the afternoon we went for a ride to [local township]. And we were making sand castles at the beach, and that was about it.

(Interview 3, Joanna)

Jack's Saturday went like this:

Jack: We played PlayStation, went for walks. Fed the lambs and cows.
Int: What were the PlayStation games that you played?
Jack: X-box. We played Spiderman, and that's about it.
Int: So you really enjoy Spiderman on X-box?
Jack: Yeah.
Int: Where did you walk to when you went for a walk with your friend?
Jack: We decided to have a wee trip to go hunting. And we just went around the yard. They live out on the side of the road, and they've got quite a big place.
Int: Do they have a farm, or bush land, or what type of land do they have?

Jack: They just have a big open area with paddocks and trees.

Int: So what were you hunting for?

Jack: Rabbits. We just used sticks and wood and string. We made bow and arrows, and sharpened sticks for spears.

Int: Did you see any signs of rabbits?

Jack: We saw rabbit holes.

(Interview 3, Jack)

Functional physical activity

Playing games and sports were by no means the only kinds of physical activities characterizing these four children's daily lives. In the latter interviews, where discussion moved away from physical activity per se, each of the children revealed numerous ways in which they move for reasons other than fun or for sport. Walking the dog, biking down to the shops to get mum's groceries, delivering pamphlets to people's letter boxes, helping nana collect the eggs, cleaning the house, feeding cows and tidying rooms were just a few of the chores the children performed, each involving physical activity, yet not in the form most surveys would get at. We provide an extended description of Jack's 'Sunday' as an illustrative example of the kinds of physical activities that are regular parts of some children's lives. We doubt that Jack's rounding up the cows and helping his father unload building materials would feature on any quantitative survey of his physical activity levels, yet consider that Jack's activities would certainly count as much as any form of deliberate exercise as evidence of being physically active.

Int: Okay, what did you do on Sunday?

Jack: We had to get up about 7 o'clock and do the cattle. We had to chase the cattle around the road.

Int: Did you have to shift them to a different paddock?

Jack: Yep. We put them in with the bull. And we had to take them around to our granny's because we don't have a bull on our farm. And then we went home.

Int: Did you all do that?

Jack: Yeah, and a friend of dad's. And then we went home, had something to eat–

Int: Did you have some breakfast before you went?

Jack: Yep. And then we went around to my granny's . . . and then we went around to our farm and picked up the tractors to take them around to my granny's farm, and got them all ready to work the paddocks, shortly.

Int: So you all helped with that as well?

Jack: No, just me, dad, and mum. And then we went home and had some lunch. Then we went up to this guy's place to pick up some boxing for the new house that we are building. It's stuff that goes around the outside so you can get your concrete even. There was lots of it so by the time we'd finished and unloaded it all, it must have been about 4 o'clock.

Int: Did all three of you help with that too?

Jack: Yep. Then we went around and picked up my brother, and went home and cooked tea.

(Interview 3, Jack)

'Just for the fun of it'

One of the discourses relatively absent in current discussions around children and physical activity is that of pleasure. As physical activity becomes increasingly commodified and linked explicitly to health outcomes and to work on one's body and oneself (Burrows and Wright 2004, 2007; Evans and Davies 2004), the notion that physical activity can be joyful, fun and that it can feel good can understandably get lost. We found much evidence of the pivotal role of fun in the young people's experiences of physical activity. We also encountered some rich descriptions of what it feels like to be doing something one enjoys. Without direct prompting, Melissa, for example, talked at some length about what it feels like to ride a horse along the beach in the sunshine, while Joanna gave a vivid account of what her body feels like when she is rollerblading around the streets of Wallacetown:

> Rollerblading is like sort of driving your car, but going much slower . . . I like the feeling where I am trying to run in them, I do all sorts . . . it's like running and walking, Your legs are lifting up and down, and you spend ages on it, and you're moving your legs, and when you are rollerblading you are lifting the heavy roller blade up and putting it back down on the ground, and you start rollerblading again, and you're pumping your legs up, like pumping your blood . . . it's fun. I like going down the hills really fast!
>
> (Interview 3, Joanna)

These evocative descriptions did *not* accompany the children's narratives about their engagement in 'sport' per se. Indeed, one of their complaints about activities like organized tennis (for Melissa) and cricket (for Jack) lessons was the 'boring' nature of the instruction and the lack of 'fun' associated with them. When Joanna was asked what she was thinking about when she swam in her local community pool, she replied 'I'm thinking about finishing, counting the lengths . . .' Joanna's mum encouraged her to swim for 'exercise' and rewarded her for swimming a specified number of lengths with a bottle of 'fizzy drink'. This response is markedly different in tone and tenor from Joanna's extended narrative about the joys of rollerblading. Similarly there was considerably less enthusiasm expressed when discussing the physical activity organized for them in school time (e.g. jump jam aerobics and running) compared to that of their own choosing in their own time.

Relationship to popularly expressed 'concerns' about young people

Given that Wallacetown primary school was part of a university-funded study designed to change children's eating habits and get them more active (the APPLE Programme), and in light of the number of health-related programmes and initiatives present in the school, we imagined the children might have had quite a bit to say about these in their interviews. We were mistaken. Each of the children was able to rattle off lists of the 'programmes' they 'do' in school. Ambulance safety (blowing into dummies mouths, says Melissa); safety-wise, fire-wise and perhaps the most memorable 'Life Education' – 'a big bus and a giraffe'. They recalled little they wanted to share about what went on in these programmes but rather remembered the 'name' of them and in the case of 'Life Education', the fact there was a giraffe called Harold that told them what healthy foods to eat and how to deal with bullying. Jack had no memory of anything he'd done about 'health' in school – indeed his response to being asked about what he learns about health was, 'How do you mean by that?'

Similarly, while we anticipated, at least from the girls, some commentary on the relationship between physical activity and losing weight, there was no explicit linking of these two phenomena in any of the children's talk. Even though many health initiatives in schools are emphasizing physical activity as a route to fitness and therefore health, children in our study rarely mentioned 'getting fit' in their responses. Apart from Joanna, who believed that rollerblading 'makes your legs fit' and that swimming was a form of 'exercise' rather than fun, each of the children were far more likely to discuss their physical activity as something that was 'fun' and a good thing to do with friends than directly link it to increased fitness.

Another popularly reiterated theme in discussions around children's physical activity levels is the increased risks and dangers to their participation posed by strangers, motorists, unsafe neighbourhoods and geographical environments (Wong 2005). However, ready access to paddocks, paths, pools, rivers, courts and other play spaces was taken for granted in these young people's stories of their engagement in physical activity. No child identified accessibility in terms of transport to venues, existence of venues or money to 'play' as an issue of much relevance for them. Nor was there any sense that their neighbourhoods or the people in their community they bumped into in their travels posed any threat to their well-being. The notion that you can hunt rabbits in the backyard, gallop along the beach on a horse, wander across the road to a swimming pool or up to nanas to feed the chickens seemed nothing out of the ordinary to them. While not wanting to feed into idealized notions of rural paradises where everything is as it once was (Nairn *et al.* 2003; Valentine 1997, 2004), the standout thing for me in talking with these young people is the divergence of their stories from those we are being told about children in general in relation to opportunities *and* tendencies to engage in physical activity. They cast new light on universalizing accounts of the 'state of our nation's youth' and indeed, on the constituents of contemporary youth culture. The 'grown up too soon', fashion-obsessed, media-savvy consumers that some commentators suggest youth have become were missing in action on the days we interviewed these youngsters. K-mart (a cheap department store) as the label of choice and 'farming' and 'horse' magazines as the top picks for teen reading do not fit with images of youth purveyed in popular culture, nor the ones health and physical activity commentators are worrying about. Of course this may all change as the children move to high school and in future research it would be helpful to re-interview these youngsters and see what sense they make of it all now they are 'big kids' at the local high school.

Conclusion

What, if anything can the stories of these four youngsters tell us, given they are just four children from one community in the back blocks of rural New Zealand? They certainly cannot give us a generalized picture of what young people are up to in terms of physical activity in New Zealand, but they do point to the utility of talking with children and endeavouring to access and understand their lives 'in the round' outside of the school gates – something Kirk (1997) and others have been urging for quite some time.

One of the most interesting things for us was seeing (in body language) and hearing (intonation and volume) the different ways in which these children regarded their in and out of school physical activity experiences. They were each more visibly enthused when talking about stuff they did in 'their own time' yet as physical educators, we often gauge our success at inculcating appropriate attitudes towards physical education from dispositions observed and recorded 'in school'. Second, physical activity conceived in its broadest sense was an integral part of their lives, whether this be functional movement (e.g. walking the dog, collecting paua, walking to school, helping nana collect the eggs from the hen house or rounding up the sheep), engagement in institutionalized games and pursuits (e.g. tennis, rugby, motocross riding), just 'playing' (chasing rabbits, making sandcastles) or taking off on a horse or to the river for a swim because it was hot. Granted, these are just four children, living in an environment where opportunities for these things abound, yet where *are* these children in the doom and gloom statistics around declining physical activity levels for young people in New Zealand? If nothing else, our analysis encourages a wariness of generalized pronouncements about the state of our nation's youth and one-size-fits-all solutions to the envisaged problem. It alerts us to the importance of regarding and assessing children's engagement in physical activity within local contexts, families and communities, contexts which differ markedly from region to region and within provinces in New Zealand. Finally, our small-scale study points to the value in recognizing and seeking to understand children as social actors, capable of articulating the nature of their experiences, recognizing the ways economic, familial, social and cultural factors influence their engagement in physical culture, reflecting on what their futures may hold and participating as young citizens in the communities within which they currently live.

In future work, interviews with parents and other family members could be useful in an effort to further understand the ways families are implicated in the production of the habitus of individuals (Torres and Arnott 1999). In each of the children's accounts, there appeared to be little disjunction between the way they conducted their lives and their family's expectations. Indeed for each of them, family dispositions seemed favourably disposed to engagement in physical activity in all its manifestations. What Bourdieu (1984) refers to as intergenerational continuities seem, at least at this early stage (i.e. 10–11 years of age), at play in the narratives of these young children. Evans (2004) has argued that physical capital is something distributed rather unevenly across school and community contexts. He and others claim that children acquire the physical resources and capital they need to engage in new discursive regimes in family and homes. If this is so, then each of the four children in the current study seem relatively well-equipped to function in a range of physical activity contexts. Not one of them expressed any sense of themselves as physically inept or lacking in capacity to move in ways that they enjoyed or needed to in order to conduct their lives in ways they wanted to. What enables this sense of themselves as physically 'OK' and what contributes to their capacity to see physical activity as something that is fun and that makes you feel good are tropes that need further enquiry. Building castles in the sand may not count as exercise on quantitative physical activity surveys yet these and other everyday activities certainly figure in the physical culture landscape for the children in our study.

Notes

1   In New Zealand's Health and Physical Education curriculum, Physical Activity is just one of seven 'key areas of learning' and Sport Studies is another. A clear distinction between physical *activity* and *sport* is drawn throughout the document with attempts to broaden the interpretation of what counts as 'physical activity'. Indeed the description accompanying the KAL 'physical activity' does not mention 'sport' at all.

References

Abbott-Chapman, J. A. and Robertson, M. E. (2002) 'Youth, leisure and home: space, place and identity', *Society and Leisure*, 24, 2: 485–506.
Abbott-Chapman, J. A. and Robertson, M. E. (2008) 'Leisure, place and identity', in A. Furlong (ed.) *International Handbook on Youth and Young Adults*, London: Routledge.
Bishop, R. and Glynn, T. (1999) *Culture Counts*, Palmerston North: Dunmore Press.
Bourdieu, P. (1984) *Distinction: a social critique of the judgement of taste*, Cambridge, MA: Harvard University Press.
Burrows, L. (1999) 'Discourse dynamics in undergraduate physical education teacher education', paper presented at the Joint AARE/NZARE Conference, Melbourne Convention Centre, Melbourne, 26 November – 3 December.
Burrows, L. and Wright, J. (2004) '"Being healthy": young New Zealanders' ideas about health', *Childrenz Issues*, 8, 1: 7–12.
—— (2007) 'Prescribing practices: shaping healthy children in schools', *International Journal of Children's Rights*, 15: 1–16.
Chen, A. (1996) 'Student interest in activities in a secondary school physical education curriculum: an analysis of student subjectivity', *Research Quarterly for Exercise and Sport*, 67, 4: 424–32.
Durie, M. (1998) *Whaiora: Māori health development*, Auckland: Oxford University Press.
Evans, J. (2004) 'Making a difference? Education and "ability" in physical education', *European Journal of Physical Education*, 10, 1: 95–108.
Evans, J. and Davies, B. (2004) 'Endnote: the embodiment of consciousness: Bernstein, health and schooling', in J. Evans, B. Davies and J. Wright (eds) *Body Knowledge and Control: studies in the sociology of physical education and health*, London and New York: Routledge.

Featherstone, M. (1991) 'The body in consumer culture', in M. Featherstone, M. Hepworth and B. Turner (eds) *The Body – Social Process and Cultural Theory*, London: Routledge.

Gard, M. (2004) 'An elephant in the room and a bridge too far, or physical education and the "obesity epidemic"', in J. Evans, B. Davies and J. Wright (eds) *Body Knowledge and Control: studies in the sociology of physical education and health*, London and New York: Routledge.

Gard, M. and Wright, J. (2005) *The 'Obesity Epidemic': science, ideology and morality*, London: Routledge.

Hancox, R. J. and Poulton, R. (2006) 'Watching television is associated with childhood obesity – but is it clinically important?', *International Journal of Obesity*, 30: 171–75.

Hills, L. (2007) 'Friendship, physicality, and physical education: an exploration of the social and embodied dynamics of girls' physical education experiences', *Sport, Education and Society*, 12, 3: 317–36.

Jenkins, K. and Ka'ai, T. (1994) 'Maori education: a cultural experience and dilemma for the state – a new direction for Maori society', in E. Coxan (ed.) *The Politics of Learning and Teaching in Aotearoa-New Zealand*, Palmerston North: Dunmore Press.

Kirk, D. (1997) 'Sociocultural research in physical and health education', in J. Wright (ed.) *Researching in Physical and Health Education*, Wollongong: University of Wollongong.

Laclau, E. and Mouffe, C. (1985) *Hegemony and Socialist Strategy: towards a radical democratic politics*, London: Verson.

MacDougall, C., Schiller, W. and Darbyshire, P. (2004) 'We have to live in the future', *Early Child Development and Care*, 17, 4: 369–87.

Martin, L. (2002) *The Invisible Table: perspectives on youth and youthwork in New Zealand*, Palmerston North: Dunmore Press.

Ministry of Education (1999) *Health and Physical Education in the New Zealand Curriculum*, Wellington: Learning Media.

Nairn, K., Panelli, R. and McCormack, J. (2003) 'Destablizing dualisms: young people's experiences of rural and urban environments', *Childhood*, 10,1: 9–42.

Peterson, C. (1996) *Looking Forward Through the Lifespan*, Upper Saddle River, NJ: Prentice-Hall.

Pope, C. C. (2006) 'Lessons from Billy Elliot', Unpublished Phillip Smithells Memorial Lecture, *ICHPER SD* Oceania Conference, Wellington, October 1–4.

Sharples, P. (2007) 'Tino Rangatiratanga: a key determinant for good health in Aotearoa', Unpublished address delivered at New Zealand Health Teachers' Association Conference 'Our Health, Our Children, Our Future', Dunedin, July 3.

Skelton, T. and Valentine, G. (eds) (1998) *Cool Places: geographies of youth cultures*, London: Routledge.

Smith, A. (2003) 'Peer relationships in physical activity contexts: a road less travelled in youth sport and exercise psychology research', *Psychology of Sport and Exercise*, 4: 25–39.

Stothart, B. (1992) 'What is physical education?', *New Zealand Journal of Health, Physical Education and Recreation*, 25, 2: 7–9.

Torres, P. and Arnott, A. (1999) 'Educating for uncertainty in a changing world: issues within an Australian remote indigenous context', *Comparative Education*, 35, 2: 225–35.

Valentine, G. (1997) 'A safe place to grow up? Parenting, perceptions of children's safety and the rural idyll', *Journal of Rural Studies*, 13, 2: 137–48.

—— (2004) *Public Space and the Culture of Childhood*, London: Ashgate.

Van den Bulck, J. (2000) 'Is television bad for your health? Behavior and body image of the adolescent "couch potato"', *Journal of Youth and Adolescence*, 29, 3: 273–88.

Williams, A. and Bedward, J. (2002) 'Understanding girls' experience of physical education: relational and situated learning', in D. Penney (ed.) *Gender and Physical Education: contemporary issues and future directions*, London: Routledge.

Wong, G. (2005) 'The cottonwool kids', *Metro*, 284: 24–30 and 32–33.

Wright, J. and Dean, R. (2007) 'A balancing act – problematising prescriptions about food and weight in school health texts', *Utbildning & Demokrati – Journal of Didactics and Educational Policy*, 16, 2: 75–94.

13 The visions, voices and moves of young 'Canadians'

Exploring diversity, subjectivity and cultural constructions of fitness and health[1]

Margaret MacNeill and Geneviève Rail

This chapter reports on a project in Canada that draws on the model of the *Life Activity Project* to investigate how young people residing in Canada[2] discursively construct fitness and health. We focus on the ways youth from diverse social and cultural locations make sense of bodily discourses and negotiate practices associated with fitness, nutrition and health. This postcolonial feminist analysis will address how young people appropriate or resist bodily discourses and constitute themselves as subjects within them. Our analysis prompts a consideration of assumptions made by health researchers, curriculum and policy makers, teachers, and youth camp leaders about the manner in which ideas about fitness and health are taken up by young Canadians, and proposes alternative ways of theorizing young people's engagement with these cultural ideas.

The school and sports/fitness-oriented summer camp are key sites where Canadian youth receive lessons and directives about transforming their individual bio-selves into 'active healthy living' citizens. The *Canadian Youth Constructions of Health and Fitness* project has included sites in the provinces of Ontario, Newfoundland, Nova Scotia and Quebec. This chapter will offer insights from youth residing in the greater Toronto and Halton areas of central Canada. Toronto is Canada's largest city and Halton is situated on the western suburban outskirts of this megapolis. The purpose of this research was: to provide a 'snapshot' of the meanings constructed about health and fitness by youth aged 13 to 15 years of age; to uncover the educational and cultural sources from which youth derive these ideas; to explore claims youth make about how they deploy these notions in their everyday lives; to question relationships between their constructions and prevailing discourses; and to observe how youth are positioned and/or participate in resisting these discourses. In the first section, we briefly overview the research contexts and methodological considerations. In the second section, we offer an overview of developments in critical health education studies of the body – particularly developments in studies of governmentality, biopolitics and biopedagogy – and then further develop this using postcolonial feminism to suggest how biopedagogies deployed in physical education and health-promotion initiatives can be retheorized. We question why so many young people are immersed in biomedical and neo-liberal discourses regarding health and fitness and hailed to oppressive and colonizing subjectivities. The third section introduces the drawings and texts from the interviews, collected as part of the study, to continue the examination of both the assemblage of dominant neo-liberal subjectivities and the struggles by youth to resist the process of Othering. In the final section, we conclude that while many young people are provisionally hailed to these dominant positions, youth constructions of health and fitness are fairly diverse and at times contradictory, and that these discursive constructions do have material effects on their bodies, relationships and communities. The core mission of the postcolonial feminism we adopt is to destabilize neo-colonial discourses (Mohanty 1988). To destabilize colonial neo-liberal discourses we offer recommendations for research, health education and public health policy, as well as offer a call for the engagement of young people in programming, policy and research initiatives.

Research context and methodological considerations

A poststructuralist perspective (Weedon 1997; Wright 2001) informed by feminist postcolonial theory (McEwan 2001; Mohanty 2003), and poststructuralist visual methodologies (Hall 1997; Rose 2001; Sturken and Cartwright 2001) are deployed in this chapter to examine the discursive relations and outcomes of youth engagements with healthist discourses. As Rail argues, a poststructuralist framework provides a platform

> for an understanding of *subjectivity* as decentred and being made possible and constituted through the already gendered, heterosexualized and racialized discourses to which one has access; as a subject, one is *interpellated* or 'hailed' (Butler 1997) by various subject positions.
>
> (Rail 2009: 143)

For Foucault, this describes subjectivization or a process within which humans come to take up subject-positions. Particular subject-positions offer the codes for individuals to know how to act, behave and perform in social practices. How do positions come to be inhabited? The answer to this question lies in the operation of power within discourse (Nixon 1997). Drawing on Michel Foucault (1980), Nixon (1997) advocates an examination of power/knowledge as a key mechanism by which individuals come to be subjected to specific discursive positions, that is, positions of agency and of identity.

To examine how young people, aged 13–15, living in Canada come to inhabit positions, this chapter draws on data collected in Toronto and Halton regarding their identities, and the beliefs and practices they associate with health and fitness. Toronto is often touted as the world's most multicultural city and is Canada's largest urban centre yet the downtown Toronto camp attracts mainly Euro- and Asian-Canadian middle-class participants, who are the children of professional and clerical workers in the downtown core (banking and retail industries, university and colleges). Initially, the researchers expected the participants at the Toronto site would be more ethno-culturally diverse than the suburban Halton site. This assumption stems from general knowledge of Halton's history as a white upper middle-class enclave in recent decades and reports such as *Vital Signs* that report Toronto to be one of the most ethno-culturally and linguistically diverse cities in the world with 150 languages being spoken (Toronto Community Foundation 2009). However, the Toronto focus groups for this project attracted 16 young women campers from predominantly Euro-Canadian heritage (n = 13 young women) or Asian-Canadian heritage (n = 3 young women). The Halton site, on the other hand, attracted a greater diversity of youth from many recent immigrant and settler generations but no one self-identifying as aboriginal. Halton participants studied for this chapter, included 42 young women and 22 young men. According to the Halton principal, students attending the school were from 65 different nations of birth. Overall, Halton is the fastest-growing urban region in Canada due to migration from Toronto where rent and property prices are higher, new immigration, refugee resettlement and the re-zoning of surrounding farmland to housing development use.

Ethical approval to conduct focus group interviews and have youth produce images were acquired from the Halton District School Board, the summer camp Director in Toronto and the University of Toronto Office of Ethics. Written parental consent and youth assent was also obtained. The participants in the study used pseudonyms of their choice in the 50 minute audio-taped focus group discussions (6–8 students per group). This pseudonym was used to label the images they drew. Semi-structured focus groups were held during lunch hour breaks in schools and camps.

Focus group discussion questions and a *Draw and Script* exercise were based on the protocol set out by the larger Canadian research team. Before the focus group questions began, students were welcomed, invited to design a name tag with their 'fake name', and to begin to draw while they waited for all participants to arrive. Simple directions were given on the *Draw and Script* sheets. On one side, the young people were requested to: 'Draw an image of a *healthy* youth', and 'Define and describe what *health* means to you'. The opposite side requested: 'Draw an image of a *fit* youth', and 'Define and describe what *fitness* means to you'. Most completed this task before the focus group questions began so they would not feel peer pressure to produce drawings in response to what they heard from peers in the focus group discussion. They were assured that there were no 'right or wrong' answers since the researchers were interested in their beliefs and visions of health and fitness. They were neither instructed to draw 'ideal' images, nor themselves as a fit or healthy teen, nor were they instructed in any manner as to the gender, ability, ethno-cultural identification of the youth they were to draw. Many chatted, ate their lunches and caught up with friends while they drew the images, thus some cross-pollination of ideas occurred in the pre-discussion banter that was unregulated by the researchers yet likely affected by the *Draw and Script* instructions and knowledge of the research purposes from their consent forms.

In examining the representations of health and fitness created by youth within institutionalized settings, we adopt the constructivist approach of Stuart Hall (1997) to analyse the texts from the interviews and drawings. Hall's constructivist approach acknowledges the social, cultural and public character of language systems – be they verbal, visual, written, etc. symbolic processes – while recent feminist (e.g. Butler 1997) and postcolonial approaches extend this to also include the performative aspects of subjectivity and the material effects of colonizing discourse. The first order narrative reading of the transcripts and *Draw and Script* texts was descriptively coded for narrative differences in descriptions of health, fitness and gender. This included deductively coding responses for categories that emerged on other sites (Rail 2009) and inductively coding for new emerging themes. For the purposes specific to the aims of this chapter, the second order reading of the transcripts and drawings delved to deeper ideological levels of subjectivification to specifically examine codes of healthism, neo-liberalism and marginalizing codes of Othering in these texts.

Interdisciplinary considerations of subjectivification

Poststructuralist approaches to feminism, postcolonialism and critical health education studies of the body crystallize as an interdisciplinary research lens for this project on the subjectivification of young people. Michel Foucault's concept of *biopower* (1984/1990) and Basil Bernstein's vision of the 'totally pedagogized society' (2001) have recently been incorporated into the notion of *biopedagogy* (Fusco 2007; Harwood 2009; Wright 2009). Canada has a national health care system which is politically supported by formal health education policy in schools and many vision statements governing youth sport, dance and fitness camps. Youth, we argue, are recruited into the political efforts to produce themselves as healthy citizens and contribute to the reduction of national medicare costs. For example, the Toronto summer campsite in this study advertised 'Welcome to Camp T . . . Our camps are designed to promote healthy active lifestyles' on their website, while the Halton school is mediated by an official policy statement for physical and health education curriculum which declares

> The primary focus of this curriculum is on helping students develop a commitment and a positive attitude to lifelong healthy active living and the capacity to live satisfying, productive lives. Healthy active living benefits both individuals and society in many ways: for example, by increasing productivity, improving morale, decreasing absenteeism, reducing health-care costs, and heightening personal satisfaction. Other benefits include improved psychological well-being, physical capacity, self-esteem, and the ability to cope with stress. The expectations within this curriculum promote healthy active living through the development of physical, social, and personal skills.
>
> (Ontario Ministry of Education and Training 1999: 2)

Biopower generally refers to mechanisms deployed to discipline individual citizens and manage wider populations. Gastaldo (1997) outlines how health education has become a constructive mechanism of control that considers bodies and whole populations to be both manageable resources and objects. Shifting from repressive practices such as quarantine towards participatory discourses of empowerment, health education shifts health practices further into the community. Biopower entails two 'lines' of power: (1) the *bio-politics* of regulating populations, and (2) the *anatomo-politics* of the human body envisioned as a machine (Foucault 1984/1990). For Gastaldo, extending social support to elderly citizens to improve the overall life expectancy of a population would be an example of the former line of power, while learning to monitor one's blood pressure to check one's heart health would be an example of the latter. Twenty years later, what Gastoldo held up as illustrations of biopower mediating the lives of seniors in Brazil can easily be held up as examples of the kinds of ideas youth in Canada are summoned to today as they begin to worry about life expectancy at younger ages due to 'obesity epidemic' rhetoric.

Biopower and studies of governmentality have been theoretically extended with the notion of biopedagogy in recent years. According to Valerie Harwood (2009: 15), 'an extensive pedagogy is aimed at us: a pedagogy of *bios*, or what can be termed "biopedagogy". This biopedagogy is premised on a conflation between *bios* and health where there is far more at stake than simply "being well".' Biopedagogy is used 'to describe the normalizing and regulating practices in schools and disseminated more widely through the web and other forms of media, which have been generated by escalating concerns over claims of global "obesity epidemic"' (Wright 2009: 1).

Biopedagogies, such as daily physical activity policies, census reports on shifting BMI trends, education policies for active living, public health '*Call to Action*' policies, *Canada Food Guides*, wellness journal exercises in schools are systems of control. They put individuals and populations under surveillance, provide instruction on health risks, oblige citizens to heed particular responsibilities and encourage constant self-monitoring. Indeed, as systems of control from instruction have become a constant mediating feature of contemporary life, society can be seen as 'totally pedagogized' (Bernstein 2001, cited in Wright 2009: 1). It is crucial to recognize these systems of control as being racialized, gendered and ableist.

The medicalizing trends mentioned previously are implicated in Othering racialized bodies and non-normative bodies. Laura Azzarito (2009: 184), for example, offers an insightful critique of fitness, fatness and whiteness: 'The fit body is a transcendent, healthy body constructed upon gendered, white ideals (Seid 1989), and pedagogised through the media and the emergence of the medical, health and fitness alliance manifest in alarmist discourses of the world-wide obesity epidemic.' Racialized minorities and poor youth, she argues, are blamed and positioned as fatter than white and middle class; assumptions about whiteness, power and the rise of corporate curriculum in the form of fitness and nutrition crusades are left unchallenged. Drawing on the work of Cheryl McEwan (2001, 2009) and other postcolonial feminist scholars and political activists, we extend the work of Azzarito by understanding postcolonialism to be a mode of critique and political intervention into the *discursive* and the *material* legacies of colonialism. McEwan and other feminist postcolonial scholars have taken western feminist approaches to task for ignoring the ethno-cultural diversity, differing historical experiences, material circumstances and intersecting oppressions facing marginalized populations (Jiwani *et al.* 2006; McEwan 2001; Mohanty 1988, 2003; Spivak 1988; Suleri 1992). To redress these shortcomings, postcolonial feminism examines the historical implications of varying forms of colonization and patriarchy, the implications of the expansion of transnational capitalism, and the implications of both for lived experiences (McEwan 2009; Mohanty 2003). Both feminist and post-colonial studies are attentive to interpellation (hailing) and to questioning the manner and extent to which cultural representations and language systems are important to the processes of producing difference, identity formation and constructing subjectivity (Ashcroft *et al.* 2000; Butler 1997; MacNeill 2009; Weedon 1997; Wright 2001). Overall, this case study aims to offer a snapshot of a wider range of the complex subject positions young people residing in Canada are hailed to.

The notion of being hailed or *interpellated* refers to a process whereby humans are called upon to recognize themselves as subjects. Coined by Louis Althusser (1971), this notion illustrates how one comes to be positioned in relation to dominant ideologies, such as capitalism, and how one comes to be complicit in one's own domination. However, Althusser's neo-Marxian conceptualization is limited by (1) a lack of vision of social change since the subject is 'always already' defined, (2) vagueness in identifying the powerful agency that summons, and (3) failing to afford individuals and networks of people with any sense of agency to resist (Sturken and Cartwright 2001). Yet Althusser's notion of interpellation still retains an intertextual usefulness for examining the 'imagery' of our symbolic order and material effects on bodies and communities. Intertexuality we argue, also should consider *intercorporality* since bodies are texts that can be read and exchanged in discursive relations that, for example, rub up against and through public health active living messages, family wellness traditions, lunch room policies, curriculum guides, online advertising, nutrition labelling on cereal boxes, etc. Thus, the concept of interpellation allows us to consider the making of meaning of health in relation to a multitude of cultural texts, broader socio-historical forces and the material circumstances of the lives of youth.

On these latter points, the Gramscian notion of hegemony can be utilized to temper Althusser's overdetermined sense of domination by inserting a sense of agency. This allows for negotiations between dominant and marginalized understandings of physical activity and health. Hegemonic interpellation helps to explain the historical stubbornness of neo-liberal narratives such as healthism (see Chapter 11) and the taken-for-grantedness of white western biomedical authority mediating school and corporatized summer camp health lessons (e.g. the *Canada Food Guide* produced by the federal government is embedded into the nutrition games played at camp that were designed by the Diary Farmers of Canada). Moreover, as a concept, hegemony offers room to account for resistance during the processes of subjectification (Sturken and Cartwright 2001). Thus, interpellation can be extended to examine both how/if youth come to be discursively summoned, contingently positioned and materialized as racialized subjects, classed subjects, dis/abled subjects, heterosexualized gendered subjects and the numerous intersections possible at a given historical juncture. We believe this research lens opens up a kaleidoscope of possible understandings, relationships and ways of being active.

Interpellation can also be reformulated to explore the possibilities of preferred, negotiated and oppositional decodings of cultural texts (Hall 1980) to help us make sense of biopedagogized subjectivification. Cultural texts – such as the body mass index, *Canada's Physical Activity Guide* and personal wellness journals – are popular devices frequently used in health education lessons in both school and summer camp settings in Canada. They serve as biopedagogical devices that can hail subjects to particular positions. The recent works of Valerie Harwood (2009) and Deana Leahy (2009) are particularly useful for theorizing this process of subjectivification. Leahy (2009: 176) suggests that knowledge is only one aspect of a 'biopedagogical assemblage' and is not a biopedagogical device in and of itself. Leahy cogently argues that the assemblance of nutritional knowledges during pedagogical work (in her case study of Australian health education classes) also requires us to enquire how these knowledges are 'folded' into how youth come to know themselves and others; how they are mobilized to perform self-monitoring and modifying behaviours; how they mobilize emotion or affect such as shame and disgust for the 'unfit body'; and how youth change or resist such pressures.

In our case study, Zhao's responses to our questions demonstrate that resistance to expert health knowledge is clearly possible in oppositional decoding of curriculum. This 14-year-old female, born into a middle-class Halton community, has parents from two different ethno-national cultures. Her mother is East-Indian descent but born in Singapore, while her father was born in Hong Kong, moved to Singapore as a teenager, and considers himself to be of 'mixed race' in calling himself 'Bombay-Chinese'. With parents working professional jobs in the banking industry in downtown Toronto, but retaining a strong sense of homeland, she proclaimed her parents possessed 'the best ideas from the east and the west about health'. Zhao may be hailed into a dominant neo-liberal position at the start of health classes that promote self-surveillance and record keeping, but she quickly conveys a discomfort with what she has learned when recounting the experience:

Int: What were the key lessons in your Grade 9 health class recently?

Zhao: Good food and lots of exercise are supposed to be the key to health. In health class, we have to keep track of everything we put in our mouth, umm, and I mean *every* morsel. Even gum has to be put in our Wellness Journal. Miss B makes us sort it into groups from the *Canada Food Guide*. We've been doing this since Grade 5. But there isn't a white stripe for gum on the Guide so it's dumb. Then we gotta figure out how many calories each group comes to, and then, umm, then see if this is more or less than what we spend on our fitness energy list. I chew sugarless so I don't even worry about it.

Int: What have these journal exercises taught you? [She becomes silent and contemplative for a few seconds, then appears frustrated].

Zhao: Dunno. My Mum makes traditional Indian makhani chicken she learned to cook at home in Singapore, but I can't put the sauce or the whole dish in one group. The rainbow of groups in the guide doesn't show all my Mum's good cookin' or healthy spices in my Didima's cupboard.

Int: What do you learn about fitness in health class?

Zhao: We just learned about burning energy, homo-something and the fitness rule. I'm also supposed to fill in the FITT formula chart[3] with activities that make my heart strong. But I do, ahh you know, Taijiquan with my Dad sometimes on the weekend. But it's so slow I don't think I burn many calories so – I can't, umm, write that in my journal.

Int: Did you learn anything about fitness or yourself from this exercise?

Zhao: Not much. Teachers don't know everything, 'cause I feel lots of energy when I move with my Dad like this [Zhao demonstrates slow circling arm motions]. My Dad says 'energy is health and health is energy'. Because how can you be, you know, healthy if you don't have energy, you know? Energy doesn't just come from moving muscles. It's not just from the right carb count or trying to burn extra fat. Health is bigger than the dumb rainbow of Canadian food. To me, umm . . . my family is a picture of health.

(Halton Focus Group 8)

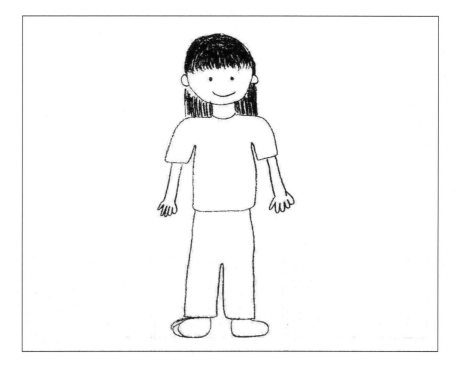

Figure 13.1 Zhao's image of 'a healthy youth'

Similar to Hall's negotiated or oppositional modes of decoding, Catherine Belsey (1980) calls this type of resistance an 'interrogative' critical reading. Despite the preferred western biophysical framework for understanding health, fitness, nutrition and energy balance are encoded into classroom lesson plans, Zhao's focus group contributions suggests she understands and practises health *relationally* and *transculturally*. She draws a simple happy smiling image of herself as young woman to depict the 'image of a healthy youth' (see Figure 13.1) yet despite rejecting the western biophysical curriculum of her school that narrowly focuses on formulae such as energy in-out caloric counting exercises to maintain 'healthy body weights', or ideas like achieving 'homeostasis' when running the school track,[4] Zhao labels her image of a 'fit youth' with tags such as 'smart and educated about health', 'healthy heart muscles', 'weights! trained fitness', 'fruits + vegetables' and 'healthy diet' (see Figure 13.2). The politics of making meaning and the active transformations that can and do occur are part of a struggle *in* discourse according to Hall (1980). To take a step further, our examination of the mediation of healthism, gender, race and other intergenerational dimensions

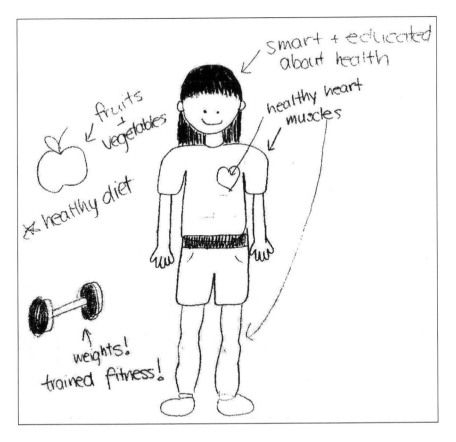

Figure 13.2 Zhao's image of 'a fit youth'

of subjectivity, suggests this struggle can also be pursued intersectionally *between* discourses.

Discursive constructions of health and fitness

When focus group participants were asked at the start of discussions, 'what does health mean to you?' and second 'what does fitness mean to you?', a similar range of initial responses were offered at both Toronto and Halton sites that confirm many observations by Geneviève Rail (2009) and Natalie Beausoleil (2009) of participants in other areas of Canada. Our first reading of the Toronto/Halton discussion transcripts, as well as *Draw and Script* sheets, involved coding for differences in health and fitness narrative themes and sorting responses by gender. Deductive narrative coding from the categories uncovered at other sites confirmed similar ranges of understandings in notions of health: being physical active (many conflate health and fitness), eating nutritiously, looking slim, having other physical qualities like good posture, avoiding bad habits, having personal qualities particularly self-esteem, being happy, feeling energetic, not being sick, having a healthy environment, having a healthy family and having good friends. Other narrative codes that have inductively emerged as we have attempted to keep our eyes open to surprises at the Toronto and Halton sites, include: health is 'not being rude', 'managing my friends' and 'a balance of mind, body and spirit'. Fitness is often described by youth as a 'capacity to do work', 'being strong in muscles and heart', 'being muscular', 'looking muscular', 'having an active goal', 'doing daily activities without getting tired', 'being good at aerobics', 'keeping up homeostasis' or 'not getting out of breath on the stairs'. The lessons of exercise physiology figure powerfully in the responses to the fitness question at both sites.

During the initial reading for health and fitness narratives, a few observations quickly emerged regarding the *Draw and Script* texts. First, not a single image of an ample, soft or fat teen was drawn to present a 'healthy teen' or the 'fit teen', despite a moderately diverse range of body shapes and sizes being present around the focus group table. Maria, for example, an ample fourth generation Italio-Canadian young woman, drew herself as a stick figure and used a pointy triangle to represent her body from neck to hips. Later in focus groups, she explained, 'Some of you may think I'm round like an apple, but I feel healthy so I don't want seem like an "apple shape" that we found out is more likely to have a heart attack when we get a little older' (Halton Focus Group 3A). Second, many participants drew a 'healthy teen' that closely resembled or caricatured themselves (particularly facial features). Third, the vast majority of images of fitness contain representations of 'six-pack' abdominal muscles, often drawn over clothes. Fourth, very few participants have drawn images that display non-white racialized facial features; however, a few young men overemphasized their hair and/or facial features as ethno-cultural markers (see Calvin's Figures 13.3 and 13.4 and the following discussion for an example of this exception). Fifth, young men were more likely to use raunchy humour and/or nude depictions as mild opposition to the exercise ('enjoyable resistance' might be a more apt description of the pleasure they took from this,

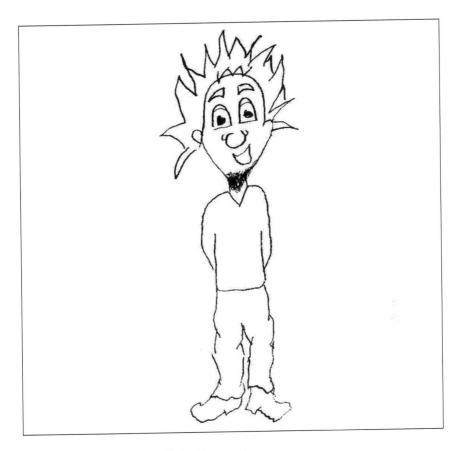

Figure 13.3 Calvin's image of 'a healthy youth'

knowing they were using pseudonyms or visual humour and teachers were not present), but they were also less likely to speak about or share their images in the focus groups. Sixth, young women often drew an image of a woman resembling themselves to depict a 'healthy teen', but about a third of all female participants drew an image of a male body to represent what a 'fit teen looks like'. Moreover, the three Muslim women who wore hijabs to the focus groups depicted male bodies as both the image of the healthy youth and the fit youth. Finally, many teens provided a list of attributes or behaviours, like a shopping list, to *describe* 'health' or 'fitness' to anchor their drawings, but about half of all participants did not articulate a definition of these terms. Perhaps this stems from notions of 'health' and 'fit' being implicated in complicated discourses that are hard to unpack.

The following focus group excerpt from a Halton Grade 10 class illustrates many of the narrative codes about health and fitness in their own words.

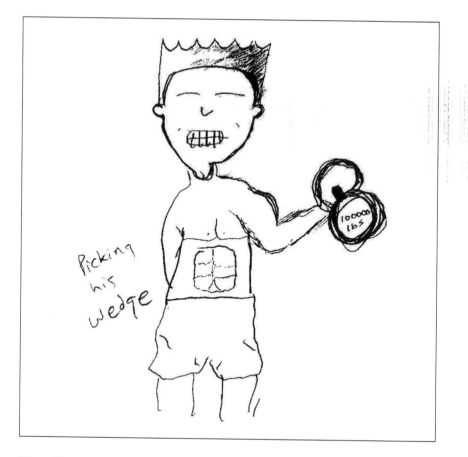

Figure 13.4 Calvin's image of 'a fit youth'

Int:	What does health mean to you?
Oprah:	I guess I think about health more than fitness. Health is feeling happy and being full of energy. I don't care if I'm fit. Health is something my Mom is always complaining needs to get back because she's always tired from work, and her back always hurts and she eats on the run. She's a nurse but she doesn't see a lot of healthy people.
Int:	Why do you care about health? Why is it important to you?
Oprah:	I think it's because my family is fat so they're all like dying. Not – like, dying, but they are always sick and everything. I worry that I am going to get sick and die off.
Int:	Is there something specific about health that you worry about?
Oprah:	No. I just try to eat healthy. We have exercise machines at my house so I try to use those.

Int: What about you Adidas? Do you care about health and what does health mean to you?

Adidas: I care about health but I don't think about it a lot really. I don't have to do anything to keep myself healthy. I kind of just stay that healthy. I never get sick. I were sick like twice in the past five years maybe.

Int: What about about fitness?

Adidas: No I don't care about fitness, I ... [interrupted].

Calvin: Bull, you care about fitness. You go all the time to the fitness studio.

Int: Calvin, what do the notions 'health' and 'fitness' mean to you?

Calvin: Well check out my fine form to find out. [He holds up a drawing of himself (see Figure 13.4)]. Health is maintaining *proper hom-eo-stasis*. Gotta balance nutrition and activity.

Adidas: Yah, then why are you standing *still* in your picture?

Gerome: Hey I'm always fit and awesome whether I'm movin' or not.

Calvin: And you haven't seen me on the finer side! [He flips over his *Draw and Script* sheet to show the fitness side and laugher erupts]. I wrote, 'fitness is having a physical goal you work for like cardio, flexibility or strength'. I'm brilliant and fit. [In the picture he is wincing his eyes as he lifts a barbell labelled '100,000 lbs' with one hand, and is loosening his shorts with the other hand. A hand written label on his fitness picture describes this as "picking his wedge".].

Adidas: That's all you can lift? You can't draw either. [Laughter] ...

Int: Do fitness and health mean different things?

Adidas: Nope. They are the same.

(Halton Focus Group 9B)

Like Oprah of American based television talk show fame, the young 'Oprah' woman, a second-generation Caribbean-Canadian, in this Halton focus group exchange, uses physical activity as a tool for getting healthier, not necessarily fitter. Many young women in this study associate fitness with slim body shape and/or the look of lean muscularity, while fitness is more of an action or physiological outcome for many males in the study. Yet Oprah stands out as one of the few young women who voices being consciously concerned with health and mortality. It may seem like a contradiction when she states 'I don't care if I'm fit' and then reveals she 'uses exercise machines at home to get healthy' and draws a slim muscular male basketball player to represent what a 'fit youth' looks like (see Figure 13.5). She is less worried about looking traditionally slim to be healthy (her image of health, see Figure 13.6, is the 'softest' body depicted in the Halton collection), than she is worried about messages that her family is at risk due to their fatness.

For most in the study, unhealthiness is something for adults to worry about. For example, the proclamation, 'I don't know what healthy is, I just am' from Smarties, a young woman who self identifies as an Irish-Canadian group figure skater from an upper middle-class neighbourhood in Toronto (Toronto Focus Group 1A), encapsulates this widespread sentiment among middle-class youth in this study on both sites who come from many ethno-cultural backgrounds, but particularly

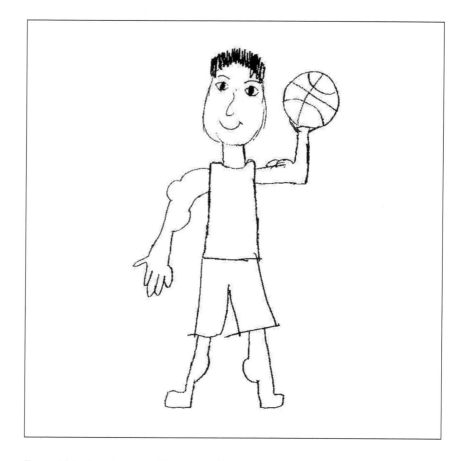

Figure 13.5 Oprah's image of 'a fit youth'

privileged Canadian western and northern eurocultures. However, the 'worry' of the few brave enough to raise these issues publicly in a focus group, suggests some of the moralizing over the obesity epidemic is having real consequences for the emotional joy and emotional health of youth, their unique conflations of health and fitness and their modifications of daily practices related to activity and eating.

We suggest that the infusion of biomedicalized knowledges into the media-rich lives of youth, as well as into the health class room, summer camp activities and, in Oprah's case, the vocational messages her Mom likely brings home from the clinical setting of hospital-based work, are sutured by youth in a manner that has real consequences for the emotional health, forms of self-care, family relations, peer interactions and political processes of Othering. As the young men in the group shifted the mood of the group away from Oprah's serious concerns for her family to the masculinist banter about megarexic muscularilty and the discomfort of gym shorts 'hurtin' your butt wedge' (Calvin, Halton Focus Group 9B), Oprah became

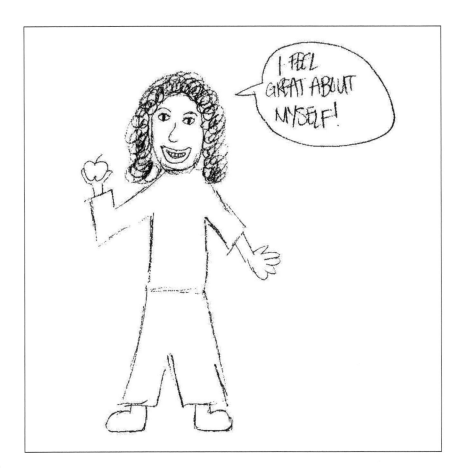

Figure 13.6 Oprah's image of 'a healthy youth'

disengaged from the rest of the conversation and returned to sketching. An ethical dilemma emerges in the paradox of trying to get at the wide range of notions of health and fitness negotiated by youth during a focus group; the discussion instigated by the researcher may reproduce dominant ideas when louder or more insistent voices are heard, thereby possibly contributing to Othering. As researchers, health promoters, physical educators, youth leaders and policy makers, we need to reconsider and redress the twin tensions of neo-liberal smothering and colonizing Othering in these discussions.

Conclusion: intercorporeal visions, voices and moves

'Contemporary dominant discourses of health and fitness strip young people's rights to make sense of their physicality through a holistic education of the body;

and function to dislodge young people from their sense of self, experiences and backgrounds' (Azzarito 2009: 193).

When we look, listen and interact with youth residing in Canada, a wide array of visions, voices and moves are revealed. Students in the secondary school system and summer sport camps are well aware of the dominant messages of neo-liberal healthism mediating curriculum and programming that they are expected to learn and enact. However, like identity, subject positioning is a slippery, complex, contingent and negotiated process. Youth can reiterate knowledges with ease and occasionally negotiate emergent or oppositional understandings. However, as health and physical activity knowledges become entangled with Eurocentric and gendered biomedical knowledges that attempt to normalize bodies, we need to continue to inquire about the meanings youth construct and the work that this entails, to question the effects, and to intervene in broader power relations of racism, sexism and slim able-bodied healthism.

Health promotion messages within physical education curriculum, municipal recreation programming and public health promotions need to *speak of* a wider range of conceptions of health that reach far beyond the current narrow biomedical focus on obesity reduction and prevention. Health knowledge circulating in institutionalized spaces can be mediated with a more diverse range of understandings held by marginalized youth – youth of size, homeless youth, youth from economically impoverished families, gay and lesbian youth, youth of differential abilities, and youth from the wide variety of cultures outside official Franco- and Anglophone eurocultures of Canada.

Still, inclusive messaging and culturally diverse curriculum alone will not be enough to foster significant shifts towards a culture of active health. To resist being hailed to colonizing neo-liberal subject positions in the current healthsphere, young people require a wider range of political advocacy strategies, programmes, resources and access to cultures of creative and pleasureable activity to achieve the rights Azzarito refers to. Some examples of initiatives currently underway emerging from this project include:

- introducing critical health and media literacy activities into the Living Schools Initiative and summer camp programmes: first, to explore beyond informational levels of literacy and develop critical and performative forms of corporeal awareness, and second, to involve students in the production of activity related e-zines and social networking sites to foster transnational discussions of health and activity at community levels;
- involving students in planning participatory action research;
- fostering peer leadership programmes that allow young women and men to develop new ideas for daily physical activity sessions within regular classroom settings that are culturally diverse and student-run; and
- engaging youth coalitions to push advocacy and policy initiatives between schools, public health, municipal parks and recreation, and other city spaces.

One example of a policy strategy that engages youth, involves a young South-Asian-Canadian woman from the Halton School, who is proposing a private member's bill into the provincial legislature with the help of the Leadership and gym class teacher and the public broadcaster. Her bill proposes that schools ensure culturally diverse and nutritious food options become available in all high school cafeterias. Her intent is not to ban or stigmatize the range of 'junk' and western foods that teens tend to consume most at school, but rather to open up a global palette of choice. This collaboration between teachers, the media and youth aims to spark both political interest in issues that matter to young people, and demonstrate the power of youth with a strong sense of agency. The bill has passed two readings in the Ontario provincial legislature.

To borrow and adapt Gail Weiss (1999) to our topic, the subjectification of youth and their embodiment of cultural discourses are always part of a process, product and intersectional game of intercorporeality; thus, an embodied ethics is needed to infuse our research, policies, activity curriculum and interactions with the young people in our midst.

Notes

1 Acknowledgements: The authors extend a special thanks to the students in Halton and Toronto for sharing their beliefs and experiences with us, as well as thank their teachers and camp leaders for facilitating our access. We thank the graduate research students from the University of Toronto – including Julie D'Aloisio, LeAnne Peterick, and Sabrina Razack – and the Social Sciences and Humanities Research Council of Canada for funding this research.
2 We neither assume that all youth residing in Canada are Canadian citizens, nor adopt an identity of 'Canadian', nor of 'hyphenated-Canadian' (such as 'French-Canadian', 'Scottish-Canadian', 'Indo-Canadian', etc.). We do this in an attempt to provisionally locate them within ethno-cultural and gendered relations. This will also allow the reader to further interrogate our assumptions stemming from our abled positions as white women scholars. It does however, raise a difficult debate we need to discuss further about celebrating the diversity and slippery-ness of multiple cultural identifications versus reproducing the decentred Other via hyphenation, which also privileges the nation in observations of subjectification (Bannerji 2000).
3 The FITT Formula is an acronym for 'frequency, intensity, time and type' of physical activity set out by the exercise physiology field. It was widely adopted since the 1970s in western fitness certification, PE curriculum and public health promotions as a cardio-respiratory prescription. It is accompanied with a clear set of rules to govern oneself (e.g. your maximum heart rate per minute for training should not exceed 220 – depending on factors such as age; Hoeger *et al.* 2009: 174).
4 According to the gym teacher, who helped to recruit participants for the study, homeostasis is a levelling off of respiratory and heart rates during moderate exercise and energy is being consistently burnt by the body.

References

Althusser, L. (1971) *Lenin and Philosophy and Other Essays*, trans. B. Brewster, London: Monthly Review Press.

Ashcroft, B., Griffiths, G. and Tiffin, H. (2000) *Post-Colonial Studies: the key concepts*, London and New York: Routledge.

Azzarito, L. (2009) 'The rise of the corporate curriculum: fatness, fitness, and whiteness', in

J. Wright and V. Harwood (eds) *Biopolitics and the 'Obesity Epidemic'*, London and New York: Routledge.

Bannerji, H. (2000) *The Dark Side of Nation: essays on multiculturalism, nationalism and gender*, Toronto: Canadian Scholar's Press.

Beausoleil, N. (2009) 'An impossible task? Preventing disordered eating in the context of the current obesity panic', in J. Wright and V. Harwood (eds) *Biopolitics and the 'Obesity Epidemic'*, London and New York: Routledge.

Belsey, C. (1980) *Critical Practice*, London: Routledge.

Bernstein, B. (2001) 'From pedagogies to knowledges', in A. Morais, I. Neves, B. Davies and H. Daniels (eds) *Towards a Sociology of Pedagogy: the contribution of Basil Bernstein to research*, New York: Peter Lang.

Butler, J. (1997) *Gender Trouble*, New York: Routledge.

Foucault, M. (1980) *Power/Knowledge*, trans. C. Gordon, L. Marshall, J. Mepham and K. Soper, Brighton, UK: Harvester Wheatsheaf.

—— (1984/1990) *The History of Sexuality, Volume I: an introduction*, London: Penguin.

Fusco, C. (2007) '"Healthification" and the promises of urban space: a textual analysis of place, activity, youth (PLAY-ing) in the city', *International Review for the Sociology of Sport*, 42(1): 43–63.

Gastaldo, D. (1997) 'Is health education good for you? Re-thinking health education through the concept of biopower', in A. Petersen and R. Bunton (eds) *Foucault, Health and Medicine*, London and New York: Routledge.

Hall, S. (1980) 'Encoding/decoding', in S. Hall, D. Hobson, A. Lowe and P. Willis (eds) *Culture, Media, Language*, London: Hutchinson.

—— (1997). 'The work of representation', in S. Hall (ed.) *Representation: cultural representations and signifying practices*, London: Sage.

Harwood, V. (2009) 'Theorizing biopedagogies', in J. Wright and V. Harwood (eds) *Biopolitics and the 'Obesity Epidemic'*, London and New York: Routledge.

Hoeger, W. W. K., Hoeger, S. A., Locke, M. and Lauzon, L. (2009) *Principles and Labs for Fitness and Wellness*, 1st Canadian Edition, Toronto: Nelson.

Jiwani, Y., Steenbergen, C. and Mitchell, C. (2006) *Girlhood: redefining the limits*, Montreal: Black Rose Books.

Leahy, D. (2009) 'Disgusting pedagogies', in J. Wright and V. Harwood (eds) *Biopolitics and the 'Obesity Epidemic'*, London and New York: Routledge.

McEwan, C. (2001) 'Postcolonialism, feminism and development: intersections and dilemmas', *Progress in Development Studies*, 1(2): 93–111.

—— (2009) *Postcolonialism and Development*, London: Routledge.

MacNeill, M. (2009) 'Opening up the gendered gaze: sport media representations of women, national identity and the racialized gaze in Canada', *Olympic Women and the Media: international perspectives*, New York: Palgrave Macmillan.

Mohanty, C. T. (1988) 'Under Western eyes: feminist scholarship and colonial discourse', *Boundary*, 2(12–13): 71–92.

—— (2003) *Feminism Without Borders: decolonizing theory, practicing solidarity*, London: Duke University Press.

Nixon, S. (1997) 'Exhibiting masculinity', in S. Hall (ed.) *Representation: cultural representations and signifying practices*, London: Sage.

Ontario Ministry of Education and Training. (1999) *Health and Physical Education: the Ontario curriculum Grades 9 and 10*, online. Available URL: http://www.edu.gov.on.ca/eng/curriculum/secondary/health910curr.pdf (accessed: 20 July 2009).

Rail, G. (2009) 'Canadian youth's discursive constructions of health in the context of the obesity discourse', in J. Wright and V. Harwood (eds) *Biopolitics and the 'Obesity Epidemic: governing bodies'*, London and New York: Routledge.

Rose, G. (2001) *Visual Methodologies*, London: Sage.

Seid, P. R. (1989) *Never Too Thin: why women are at war with their bodies*, London: Prentice Hall.

Spivak, G. (1988) 'Can the Subaltern speak?', in C. Nelson and L. Grossberg (eds) *Marxism and the Interpretation of Culture*, Urbana, IL: University of Illinois Press.

Sturken, M. and Cartwright, L. (2001) *Practices of Looking: an introduction to visual culture*, New York: Oxford University Press.

Suleri, S. (1992) 'Women skin deep: feminism and the postcolonial condition', *Critical Inquiry*, 18(4): 756–69.

Toronto Community Foundation (2009) *Vital Signs Report 2009*, online. Available URL: http://www.tcf.ca/vitalinitiatives/TVS09FullReport.pdf (accessed: 30 October 2009).

Weedon, C. (1997) *Feminist Practice and Poststructuralist Theory*, London: Blackwell.

Weiss, G. (1999) *Body Images: embodiment as intercorporeality*, New York and London: Routledge.

Wright, J. (2001) 'Gender reform in physical education: a poststructuralist perspective', *Journal of Physical Education New Zealand*, 34(1): 15–25.

—— (2009) 'Biopower, biopedagogies and the obesity epidemic', in J. Wright and V. Harwood (eds) *Biopolitics and the 'Obesity Epidemic'*, London and New York: Routledge.

Part IV
Methodological issues

Showing respect

14 Reflections on methodological issues

Lessons learned from the *Life Activity* projects

Jan Wright, Doune Macdonald, Lisette Burrows, Matthew Atencio, Kelly Knez, Judy Laverty, Jessica Lee, Alison Nelson, Gabrielle O'Flynn and Bonnie Pang

In this concluding chapter, we offer some reflections on the conduct of our research that we believe have relevance across most qualitative studies that involve young people, particularly young people from diverse social and cultural groups. In the case of the *Life Activity Project* and related studies, we also needed to attend to the added sensitivity associated with researching young people's meanings of health and, inevitably, their feelings and thoughts about their bodies and body weight. What follows are some stories, dilemmas and reflections 'from the field'. The contributors to the book share issues around: recruiting participants to the research process and maintaining participants' involvement; developing respectful relationships; and, the dilemmas of researching Others and representing their voices. These reflections come from fieldnotes, thesis manuscripts and contributors' input into our closing discussions on methodological issues. In many cases these have been included as verbatim quotes.

The *Life Activity Project* was motivated by questions such as: how have family, community and school-based experiences shaped, and continue to shape, young people's current understandings and choices of physical activity; how have physical activity and physical culture provided resources for the ways in which young people constitute their identities; on what sources of meanings do they draw to construct their notions of health; and, how do their understandings of health, in turn, influence the choices they make in relation to physical activity? Projects that budded off from, or were influenced by, the original project took all or some of these questions as their focus in relation to particular groups of young people, circumscribed by a common social or cultural location such as those defined by place (e.g. rural and remote; urban), socio-economic status, or ethnicity (Indigenous; Hong Kong Chinese; African American).

In a social context in which young people are often positioned as a 'problem', all contributors to this book were keen to reflect on what we as individual researchers bring to the research process, how we position ourselves within it and how we understand and speak about our research participants. As others such as Stephen and Squires (2003) and McLeod and Malone (2000) point out, significant effort is needed to represent the meanings, constructions, values and imperatives that each individual young person works with, without further problematizing young people's engagements.

> It is clearly incumbent on us all as youth researchers neither to portray so-called 'deviant' young people as victims or dupes to structure or to erroneously celebrate them as completely free actors for our own ideological ends. We must simply listen to what young people themselves have to say when making sense of their own lives.
>
> (Stephen and Squires 2003: 161)

All of the authors in this collection were very much aware of the researcher/researched relationship and issues with subsequent representations. In all of the chapters in the book we have, we hope, acknowledged that as researchers we:

> cannot hide behind the mask of objectivity and pretend that [we] are not inti-mately involved in the research that [we] do. . . . If researchers continually remove reference to the realities of the research process from their writings, the difficulties associated with doing research, particularly on sensitive topics, are likely to remain hidden.
>
> (Dickson-Swift *et al.* 2008: 22–23)

Much has been written about these ethical issues, much of it in instructional terms. In this chapter through sharing researchers' reflections on their experiences, we attempt to take up this challenge and make visible at least some of the 'realities' of doing research with young people.

Recruiting participants

Recruitment of participants to the various studies was not always easy. For the *Life Activity Project* in Australia, the original cohort was recruited via the demographic information and responses to questions about participation in physical activity and physical education in the survey (see Chapter 1). The intention was to thereby obtain a diverse cohort of young people across a range of geographical, social and cultural locations and with differing orientations to physical activity. In addition, this first cohort was limited by those for whom their parents had consented, in the first place to the survey (positive consent was required in most states) and then to an initial interview. This was a significant limiting factor, which already moved the cohort towards young people whose parents responded to such requests and to young people who were willing to speak to those who, at this stage, were a rela-tively anonymous group of researchers. Arguably, and on the evidence of the cohort that we interviewed for the first biographical interview, this tended to mean that young people from more marginalized groups, from ethnic minorities and young Indigenous people did not volunteer. We suspect that we also were more likely to recruit those who were more confident about their activity participation and perhaps their bodies, than those who were not.

The recruitment of the longitudinal cohort from these first biographical interviews was more straightforward, since the researchers had already established contact, and hopefully established some kind of positive relationship. We were also able to select on the basis of an interview that provided us with substantially more information about the young people's life patterns of physical activity, attitudes and interests, and social and cultural contexts. The young people recruited by these means have in the main stayed with us throughout the six years of the project. The role of doctoral students has been crucial to the sustainability of the project, establishing close relationships with the participants (see the following paragraphs for some issues associated with this), and recruiting amongst those groups that might otherwise have been absent from the project. This is not to say that our recruitment covered all groups, nor that the young people we interviewed were representative of any social or cultural group – rather they provided 'windows' to the possible lives of young people who have particular social and cultural characteristics. Their everyday lives demonstrate the dangers of generalizing or making inferences from population statistics that homogenize and universalize the experiences of young people and attempt to explain their participation in physical activity simply in relation to social determinants.

In other countries, different ethics requirements, different ways of organizing the data collection and different modes of recruitment shaped the directions of the projects and the issues that were faced. For example, Amy Ha and Bonnie Pang suggest that recruitment in Hong Kong was relatively straightforward. This was for a number of reasons including: ready access to schools based upon longstanding relationships with senior staff in the schools; and, the preparedness of parents and their children to support research projects initiated by the university as a show of respect. In this case and in the case of Lisette Burrows' study of young people in New Zealand, the schools' co-operation also extended to the teachers selecting children and young people to participate in the research from those who volunteered. This prompted questions about how students were selected and for what reasons. Lisette and Bonnie respond to this dilemma:

> I guess [the teacher's] intimate knowledge of the students and their families allowed her to choose students for whom consent could be readily gained and also those who may have something to say. Inevitably this means that access to 'hard to reach' young people was effectively chopped, but given the exigencies of time, money etc. seemed like a good idea at the time. The students she selected were from different kinds of families in terms of ethnicity and socioeconomic index. [I] was happy with her choice.
>
> (Lisette Burrows)

This process of sampling students may result in teachers selecting those students who seem to be more cooperative and whose parents are not easily offended. This might have created a narrower representation of voice, in which the student might be the 'better' ones at schools. One suggestion for further research is that we could also interview the teachers to understand the reasons of their choice of particular students.

(Bonnie Pang)

In hoping to work with urban, Indigenous young people, Alison Nelson also found her longstanding professional relationship with the school with which she worked critical to her initial access.

Throughout the research project, Alison continued a dual role as researcher and practitioner within the school context, although her professional practice was with younger children in the school. This was important for three reasons. First, she was able to use the connections with other family members (younger siblings, parents and grandparents working in the school), established through her professional role, to develop relationships with the young people in her research. She felt it often put young people at ease if she mentioned having seen a younger sibling that morning or a conversation she had with 'Nan'. Second, the relationships she developed with staff members and family members working in the school enabled her to follow through with interviews with young people when they left the school as 'someone would usually know someone who knew where he/she had gone'. These connections also enabled her to 'verify' certain information provided in interviews when family situations appeared complex or content was 'far-fetched'. Of course, care needed to be taken in these instances to keep interview information confidential. Finally, it was important to Alison and to the school community that she continued to 'give something back' by way of a professional service rather than just 'taking' in the form of recruiting research participants. In the time that Alison was researching in the school, another research project took place and staff frequently pointed out the lack of ongoing input or contact from this researcher once he had his data.

The socio-political climate during which Kelly Knez's research was conducted had a significant impact upon the recruitment of young people to her project. The world had recently witnessed the September 11 bombings, the Bali Bombings in which a number of Australians were killed, the invasion of Iraq by the 'coalition of the willing' and a number of home raids on Muslim families by Australian secret service police. After an unsuccessful attempt to recruit participants from a local Islamic school, she was able to speak with a group of young Muslim women from a local state high school. When talking to the group about their potential participation, she stressed that they would remain anonymous, the irrelevance of whether they liked or disliked physical activity, and the importance of having young Muslim women from different cultural and family backgrounds in the study.

Developing relationships

After several interviews, relationships with the young people also became important, with some young people commenting that they enjoyed spending time talking with me (e.g. 'You're nice. I get along [with you], I enjoy coming here, I don't mind you recording me or nothing. It's nothing big to me' (Jacinta)) and, as trust and familiarity were developed, some young people began to speak more freely and offer more information. I tended towards also offering information about myself and my family and I think this helped build that relationship.

(Alison Nelson)

Many of the projects relied on speaking with the young people over an extended period of time, up to five years in some instances. This commitment from the participants often rested on a good relationship with the researchers conducting the interviews. At the same time the level of rapport developed between the researcher and participant had an impact on their self-thinking, their reflexivity about their lives and their desire, it could be said, to become 'better' (more active) citizens. It is not surprising that the following excerpt comes from Faye, a student from the elite girls school, where a high degree of reflexivity was evident in much of their talk about their lives (see also Chapters 5, 10). When asked how she felt about participating in the research, Faye replied:

I thought it was a different idea when I first heard about it, it's not something I've actually heard of being done. No, I think it's interesting, I think it's an interesting thing to look at, not necessarily easy though because there's so many aspects that you have to look at and I think it's actually a pretty hard thing to look at. It's funny I think it's been a pretty good experience because I think when I first started out it was like doing things like the journal . . . I think that actually made me want to do more physical activity; yeah so I think during that year, or two years, yeah, we felt like just doing more physical activity because of the fact that you were being like monitored. It was a good thing I think, I mean it was partly the reason why we did it, yeah. So I thought that was pretty funny.

(Faye, interview 2003)

A number of young people interviewed in the *Life Activity Project* (and the associated Laverty study as well) talked about the interview process as something they looked forward to. For example, Tomiko (from Bloomsbury High School) described how she felt able to discuss aspects of her life that she had not, and would not necessarily, share with others, including close friends. Gabrielle writes in her fieldnotes how Tomiko 'described how she would make a mental note about an event or involvement that she wanted to share as part of the next interview'.

Gabrielle: How have you felt about participating in general?
Tomiko: Good, yes; I don't know if it's making an impact. I really like doing it. In a way it's good to talk to someone – like not my family and not like my usual friends – but I can just tell you about my life at the moment and I find it good to talk about that. But I don't know whether I'm a really good person for your research because I don't know whether you pick lots of sporty people but I'm like one of the non-sporting people and I'm doing your research, so I feel like . . .

Gabrielle: No, why do you feel like that? Do you feel a bit guilty or something?

Tomiko: I don't know whether I'm giving you any information because I'm not doing much at all. I don't know, it's nice to do something else, like this is another one of my, something else apart from the Con [Conservatorium], yeah, I like it.

(Tomiko, interview 2002)

In Judy Laverty's study, each young person indicated it was helpful having someone who listened to them and gave them the opportunity to reflect on their lives and their various achievements and issues at regular intervals. For example, Katrina in her third interview with Judy stated: 'I wouldn't really think about things I've done, it feels good to look back over the last year or so'. This seems to respond to Scheurich's (1997) comment that the interview process is a form of chaos/freedom, where people's emotional needs or desire to communicate are being satisfied through these interactions. And young people are not powerless in the data collection process. As suggested by Scheurich (1997: 71):

> Interviewees do not simply go along with the researcher's program, even if it is a structured rather than open one. I find that interviewees carve out space of their own, that they can often control some or part of the interview, that they push against or resist my goals, my intentions, my questions, my meanings.

In relation to this, Kelly writes of the young women in her study:

> forgetting [to attend] interviews, wanting to be interviewed in pairs with a friend rather than individually, purposefully talking at length to each question so the interview would run overtime and into the next lesson, not wanting to talk about physical activity . . . and sometimes their resistance was silence.

(Kelly Knez)

And at times, the young people withdrew from the research:

> One of these students disengaged from formal schooling during the project and, despite informal contact (she lived in my local area), she appeared reluctant to continue interviews. If I had pursued this she probably would have agreed to be interviewed but I sensed a reluctance and needed to trust my 'reading' of the situation.

(Alison Nelson)

In another example, Gabrielle, writes about the ways she felt distinctly uncomfortable when Karin began questioning her, including asking her questions about her own eating habits and asked her 'how she stayed skinny?' In the following quote from a paper Gabrielle wrote on the power relation in the interview process, she reflects on this phenomenon.

In addition to this, Karin, on occasions, asked me questions. In doing so, and often to my surprise, she challenged the interviewer/interviewee power relations. Some of these questions involved Karin asking me about the sports I played and if I had a 'boy friend'. Other times, she threw me off guard and asked about my 'health' practices and body. During the health interview, for example, after talking about why she wouldn't want to put anymore weight on, Karin asked me – 'How do you stay so skinny?' – a question which shifted the interview dynamic and which was permitted by discourses around femininity and health. It seems that, through reading my body shape and size, Karin made an assumption about my position in relation to the weight loss and 'ideal' thin feminine body discourse. She seems to assume that I share her position in relation to these discourses. I recall feeling uncomfortable in taking up this shared position both because of my position as the interviewer and as a young woman who is invested in taking a critical position in relation to such discourses around femininity, health and the body. I was completely baffled as to how to answer her question, and resorted to, what I thought could only be an 'impartial' answer, shyly stating: 'It must be my metabolism.' At the time, this answer seemed 'impartial' because it rested on a rationality of genetics and so, positioned my body and practices as being outside of Karin's strict investment into weight loss practices. It was also an answer which Karin was not looking for. She wanted me to share my 'secrets' with her. So, by resorting to an answer which explained my body in terms of biology, I quickly shut down the conversation. Interestingly, if I was asked the same question, by some one outside of the interview context, I would probably resort to a modest reply and say: 'I'm not skinny.'

(O'Flynn 2004: 131)

Gabrielle also wrote about how her interviews (and the same could be said for all of the researchers) became a potential site encouraging the very 'practices for engaging with the self, including self-examination and self-monitoring' that we were concerned to critique in relation to dominant discourses of health.

My concern for seeing the interviews in this way emerged through my observations of the young women engaging with the interviews as a site through which they monitored their practices and lives. This was most prominent when I telephoned the young women to arrange an interview time. Some of the young women, for example, responded with comments, such as 'But I haven't done much physical activity lately' or 'But, I've been so lazy'. I also became aware of the ways in which the interviews were a site through which the young women and myself engaged in a particular kind of 'talk' as young women. These ways of talking and engaging seem to be located in a discourse of friendship and resulted in the interviewee/interviewer relations being inseparable from relations of trust, laughter and solidarity. My concerns do not lie with the development of 'biasing' friendships with participations. My concerns, instead, stem from my ability to draw upon a discourse of friendship to create an interview context which encouraged the young women to talk at length about themselves. This was, and remains, problematic for me because the more the young women talked about their meanings of health and physical activity, the more they examined their lives in relation to what I view as problematic meanings of health.

(O'Flynn 2004: 123)

Such dilemmas have been flagged by Foucault in his writings related to the 'pastoral power' of the interview act and the potential harmful impact on the participant (Toll and Crumpler 2004). Foucault maintained that particular types of power circulate in the caring for others, a relationship that can be generated through the interview process as the interviewer seeks to save, look after and come to know the interviewee. However, argued by Dickson-Swift *et al.* (2008), relatively little attention has been paid to the emotional and physical safety of the researcher. For example, Judy Laverty wrote in her fieldnotes:

I hadn't really thought through how affected I would be by these conversations [with young participants]. I've worked in many different communities and seen some tough stuff, but this was different. I felt rattled by the trauma [who wouldn't be?], guilty about how good my life was, angry about a care system that had failed these young people and yet blown away by each person's resourcefulness in getting by so far. While roles and responsibilities of researchers can be drilled into you, you can never be fully prepared for what will happen in an interview and how you will process this. This group of young people had seen many, many professionals come and go in their lives – social workers, care workers, foster carers etc. While I tortured myself about being another one, I realized the best I could do as a researcher was to stay honest, be up front (for example, about how long I would be around), always turn up when I said I would and genuinely listen to what they were saying. Listening seemed to be the way I could 'give back'.

(Laverty, fieldnotes May 2006)

Researching others

The delimiting of the number of participants whom the researchers sought to 'know' often involved identifying a group of young people based upon a perceived shared characteristic such as geographical location, ethnicity or socio-economic status. In doing so, it may have been that our 'practices of naming and knowledge construction den(ied) all autonomy to those so named and imagined, extending power, control, authority, and domination over them' (Goldberg 2009: 227). Those researchers working with young people from 'minority' ethnicities were particularly sensitive to working with Others with the concomitant 'traps' of claiming to 'know what is best for the Other . . . existentially, politically, economically, culturally' (Goldberg 2009: 227). Alison Nelson reflects on this issue in relation to her study with Indigenous young people.

One of the observations I have made in this project has been the importance of identifying Indigenous people as a group to work with precisely to identify the intra-group diversity and the ways in which this group of young people are the same and different to myself, non-Indigenous young people and other Indigenous young people. In other words it highlights the tenuous nature of identifying a group of people based on 'race' or 'ethnicity' or 'culture' in an urban Australian context. It also helped to highlight my taken-for-granted assumptions about being a non-Indigenous Australian but also ideas I had about Indigenous people although I had worked with Indigenous people for over 10 years. This included discovering the ways in which I (and much of policy and media around Indigenous young people) can use 'culture' as a disciplining concept (see Nakata 2007).

Ultimately this project became an opportunity to explore the ways in which the young people engaged with, disrupted, resisted and re-created discourses about both health and physical activity and about Indigenous people. As Nakata (2007: 178) notes, 'the imposition of disciplinary and disciplining standards calls in the Islander (and Aboriginal person) to measure herself/himself against the new public knowledge'. This project aimed to give an opportunity for Indigenous young people to resist this form of measurement and to offer new presentations of themselves. However, it was not without its tensions. Even bringing these assumptions to the fore of discussions was awkward and unsettling at times.

(Nelson forthcoming)

As Alison noted in her fieldnotes:

I felt so racist bringing up race in these questions today. I felt I needed to ask them but there just doesn't seem to be a 'right' way to ask about race or cultural heritage without feeling like I'm needing to make a disclaimer at the same time: 'Oh I'm not asking because I'm racist – I'm really a nice person' I feel like saying. Perhaps this discomfort is because I feel like I'm being mis-read. No wonder Aboriginal people resist the potential to be mis-read as well.

(Nelson, fieldnotes 4 November 2008)

Matthew Atencio had also to negotiate issues of race – his own and those of his participants in his study of young people in an urban neighbourhood in the United States. Matthew describes himself as an 'athlete from a minority background' ('mixed' Korean-American and Hispanic-American). The young men in his study however, despite his living in the neighbourhood for much of the time of the study, came to view him as an 'outsider'. In his reflection for this chapter he writes:

For instance, during the interviews about basketball with the African American young men, my semi-professional football background seemed to garner a certain degree of respect and friendship since they mutually understood training regimens and competition. Yet, I often came away from the interviews feeling as if their responses were indicative of boredom or even out-right disinterest. It was as if my 'mixed' background provided them with a sense of uncertainty, even though we both shared an understanding of minority 'ethnic' sport cultures. I came away from the interviews with these young men feeling like they had enacted behaviors such as acting 'cool' and disinterested (Majors and Bilson 1992). In comparison, I felt that the young 'black' women were more open and reflective. My Asian and Latino identity was quite distinct from theirs; however, my presence seemed to be read as 'non-threatening' and was conducive to their discussions about their personal lives. In these talks the young women often commented that it was their 'black' male peers who most often othered and harassed them in public spaces. Like the young women in Gabe's study, they sometimes asked me questions about my own personal relationships. Two Haitian young women, in particular, would often talk about 'fixing' me up with one of their friends and even suggested that I needed to call *them* on a more regular basis.

(Matthew Atencio)

Representation – what can we claim to know?

We are very appreciative of the time and insights given to us by the young people who participated in the projects introduced in this book. The authors attempted to tell the young people's stories in ways that are engaging. As Woolcott (1994: 17) suggests: 'Qualitative researchers need to be storytellers . . . When we cannot engage others to read our stories – our completed and complete accounts – then our efforts at descriptive research are for naught.'

Presenting the stories of others, however, is not simply about telling a good story. The authors who have contributed to this book have tried not to take the stance of those who present the 'truth'; rather, in their writing and publishing, they have often struggled with issues of presentation. Their research journeys, and eventuating stories, have been enriched (and perhaps at times burdened) by such self-reflection.

> Self-reflection has been an important process both in my reflection on my interpretation of data and reflection on anti-racist/postcolonial writings and how my analysis is influenced by my own context. It has also been vital to have Indigenous and non-Indigenous mentors who have questioned my assumptions and challenged me to wrestle with my discomforts as a white, western woman. Often these people have been a source of reassurance that my methods and approach are 'trusted' by them.
>
> (Alison Nelson)

As Alison wrote in her fieldnotes:

> This week has been a big week of dilemma regarding my role as a white researcher/representative of colonizing people. I needed to contact Vern to

both ask for advice and appease my guilt to some extent ... It strikes me that he and Pat are a reference point in all of this. So long as I feel they think it's OK, then I'm relatively confident in what I'm doing. I'm so grateful for their trust in me.

(Nelson, fieldnotes 19 November 2008)

In working with young Muslim women, Kelly Knez recounts that she is still unsettled around questions of representation:

I still haven't resolved this one in my mind, even now that I am living in the Middle East. It is hard to look beyond my 31 years of living in a western culture which has constructed Muslim women as oppressed and western ways of knowing superior, although my daily interactions with Muslim women are providing me with alternative storylines which are able to stand up against those told in the 'West'.

During my PhD I was acutely aware of this from the onset. During interviews I was cognizant of my position and made efforts to be inquisitive rather than judgmental in my questioning. During write up I included, whereever possible, long sets of data, so the reader could understand how questions were asked, answers received, and stories developed. I also purposefully avoided positioning the women as either 'oppressed' or 'free'. Did I avoid judgment? I hope so, but if not, then the way in which the data has been presented allows the reader to make their own understandings. It also allows the young women's voices to stand alone from my own interpretations.

(Kelly Knez)

Lisette Burrows recalls the 'catch 22' in the interpretation and representation of data when working with Maori and Pacifika young people:

We had one Maori young person in the small cohort – his testimony indicated a significant privileging of family relationships over 'self' in terms of his interests in physical activity, sport etc. He demonstrated a reluctance to talk about his *own* interests, proclivities, dispositions but was more visibly animated when talking about things his family did together – sociality – the collective – were paramount for him. It is easy (as I did) to presume these inclinations are a matter of cultural preference as multiple academic treatises on Maoridom emphasize this tendency to put family first, celebrate the 'group' rather than the 'individual', reluctance to talk about self – the danger in analysis is presuming this young boys' testimony *is* influenced by cultural preference when, in reality, I know nothing about the intricacies of his home life, whether or not he and his family live with Maori values and so on ... that is, it is easy to universalize the experience of ethnic groups when it could be that this young boy, like others, presumably, just 'happened' to like hanging out with his family regardless of cultural context.

(Lisette Burrows)

The issues around representation in qualitative research are not new and much debated (for example, Tierney and Lincoln 1997). For the moment we can only say that we are still grappling with these issues. A major motivation for the research was to provide the space for young people's talk about their ideas and experience of physical activity in ways that were rarely represented in the literature on youth and physical activity, which has tended, in the main, to take a deficit view of young people. A laudable aim, but we were still left with the difficult issue of how to do this: how as adults we were to represent the voices of the young people we interviewed in ways which were respectful and acknowledged their interpretations of their lives? On the other hand, inevitably and appropriately, our research voice is the one that interprets, displays the meanings derived from what the young people say to us. Whether or not the young people would recognize themselves, or their testimony in our 'tales', is another matter.

There are a number of approaches to the presentation of participants' 'voices' suggested in the literature, some of which have been taken up in the chapters in this book and some described earlier. For example, where possible we tend to provide lengthy verbatim quotes, we have tried to situate these quotes in the context of young people's lives and in the context of the interviews. In Laverty's (2008) study young people's perspectives were given a central place in the research discussion, with the research reporting focused on young people's negotiation of difficult economic and social circumstances, rather than seeking to define each young person by their disadvantage.

Other possibilities as yet not taken up are dual representations of researcher's voice alongside young person's voice where different 'readings' or interpretations are provided of their testimony within an article or chapter or the co-construction of narratives (Garrett 2004). Neither of these were strategies that we had the time or resources to do for these projects. At the same time, we are also aware that no matter what strategies we adopted in the telling of tales, the fictions/truths, we or our participants tell on any one day, are not necessarily those of tomorrow; thus locating the 'authentic' young person's voice will be a perennial (impossible) challenge. An important starting point, however, is recognizing our responsibilities as researchers and being constantly sensitive to these in the practice of our research and its presentation. As Diane Wood writes in her review of Tierney and Lincoln's (1997) book, *Representation and the Text*:

> For the postmodern researcher there is no longer a place to hide. The researcher can hide behind neither the mystification of official knowledge, the aura of the expert, the illusion of objective distance, the wordplay of language, nor the formulas of analytic logic. Not only must researchers doubt, they must do so in public by disclosing the ambiguities, contradictions, partialities, and uncertainties in their work.
>
> (Wood 1999: 390)

References

Dickson-Swift, V., James, E. and Laimputtong, P. (2008) *Understanding Sensitive Research*, Cambridge: Cambridge University Press.

Garrett, R. (2004) 'Gendered bodies and physical identities', in J. Evans, B. Davies and J. Wright (eds) *Body Knowledge and Control: studies in the sociology of physical education and sport*, London and New York: Routledge.

Goldberg, D. (2009) 'Racial knowledge', in L. Back and J. Solomos (eds) *Theories of Race and Racism: a reader*, London: Routledge.

Laverty, J. (2008) *Finding Social Relevance: young people, wellbeing and regulated support*, Doctoral Thesis, University of Wollongong. online. Available URL: http://ro.uow.edu.au/theses/128/ [Accessed: 3 February 2010].

McLeod, J. and Malone, K. (eds) (2000) *Researching Youth*, Hobart, Australia: Australian Clearinghouse for Youth Studies.

Majors, R. and Bilson, J. (1992) *Cool Pose: the dilemmas of black manhood in America*, New York: Lexington Books.

Nakata, M. (2007) *Disciplining the Savages: savaging the disciplines*, Canberra: Aboriginal Studies Press.

Nelson, A. (forthcoming) '"I do stay healthy": the meaning and place of health and physical activity in the lives of urban Indigenous young people', Doctoral Thesis, University of Queensland, Brisbane, Australia.

O'Flynn, G. (2004) 'A poststructural reflection on interviewing young women about health and physical activity', in J. Wright (ed.) *Researching in Physical and Health Education*, Wollongong: Faculty of Education, Wollongong University.

Scheurich, J. (1997) *Research Method in the Postmodern*, London: Falmer Press.

Stephen, D. E. and Squires, P. A. (2003) '"Adults don't realize how sheltered they are": a contribution to the debate on youth transitions from some voices on the margins', *Journal of Youth Studies*, 6(2): 145–64.

Tierney, W. G. and Lincoln, Y. S. (1997) *Representation and the Text: reframing the narrative voice*, Albany: State University of New York Press.

Toll, C. and Crumpler, T. (2004) 'Everything is dangerous: pastoral power and university researchers conducting interviews', in B. Baker and K. Heyning (eds) *Dangerous Coagulations? The uses of Foucault in the study of education*, New York: Peter Lang.

Wolcott, H. (1994) *Transforming Qualitative Data*, London: Sage.

Wood, D. (1999) 'Representation and the text: reframing the narrative voice', *Anthropology and Education Quarterly*, 30(3): 389–91.

Index